Overcoming Common Problems

TREATING ARTHRITIS
EXERCISE BOOK

Margaret Hills and
Janet Horwood

sheldon PRESS

First published in Great Britain in 1994

Sheldon Press
36 Causton Street
London SW1P 4ST
www.sheldonpress.co.uk

Reprinted five times
Reissued 2011

British Library Cataloguing-in-Publication Data
A catalogue record for this book is available from the British Library

ISBN 978–1–84709–161–1

1 3 5 7 9 10 8 6 4 2

Printed in Great Britain by Ashford Colour Press

Produced on paper from sustainable forests

TREATING ARTHRITIS EXERCISE BOOK

The late MARGARET HILLS SRN, trained at St. Stephen's Hospital in London, until her training was cut short by crippling heart disease and arthritis. Against all the odds she fought back and went on to marry, have eight children and pursue a long career as an industrial nurse. She developed her own method of natural treatment for arthritis, and in 1982 she opened a clinic in Coventry. She wrote several best-selling books based on her experience and success. They were *Treating Arthritis – The Drug-Free Way*, *Treating Arthritis: More ways to a drug-free life* and *Treating Arthritis Diet Book* all published by Sheldon Press.

JANET HORWOOD is health editor of *Woman's Weekly* magazine and has a particular interest in health matters. She is the author of several books including *Comfort for Depression* (Sheldon 1988). She is married with three children and lives in Kent.

Overcoming Common Problems Series

Selected titles

A full list of titles is available from Sheldon Press,
36 Causton Street, London SW1P 4ST and on our website at
www.sheldonpress.co.uk

101 Questions to Ask Your Doctor
Dr Tom Smith

Asperger Syndrome in Adults
Dr Ruth Searle

The Assertiveness Handbook
Mary Hartley

Assertiveness: Step by step
Dr Windy Dryden and Daniel Constantinou

Backache: What you need to know
Dr David Delvin

Body Language: What you need to know
David Cohen

Bulimia, Binge-eating and their Treatment
Professor J. Hubert Lacey, Dr Bryony Bamford
and Amy Brown

The Cancer Survivor's Handbook
Dr Terry Priestman

The Chronic Pain Diet Book
Neville Shone

Cider Vinegar
Margaret Hills

Coeliac Disease: What you need to know
Alex Gazzola

Confidence Works
Gladeana McMahon

Coping Successfully with Pain
Neville Shone

Coping Successfully with Prostate Cancer
Dr Tom Smith

Coping Successfully with Psoriasis
Christine Craggs-Hinton

Coping Successfully with Ulcerative Colitis
Peter Cartwright

Coping Successfully with Varicose Veins
Christine Craggs-Hinton

Coping Successfully with Your Hiatus Hernia
Dr Tom Smith

Coping Successfully with Your Irritable Bowel
Rosemary Nicol

Coping When Your Child Has Cerebral Palsy
Jill Eckersley

Coping with Age-related Memory Loss
Dr Tom Smith

**Coping with Birth Trauma and Postnatal
Depression**
Lucy Jolin

Coping with Bowel Cancer
Dr Tom Smith

Coping with Bronchitis and Emphysema
Dr Tom Smith

Coping with Candida
Shirley Trickett

Coping with Chemotherapy
Dr Terry Priestman

Coping with Chronic Fatigue
Trudie Chalder

Coping with Coeliac Disease
Karen Brody

Coping with Compulsive Eating
Dr Ruth Searle

**Coping with Diabetes in Childhood
and Adolescence**
Dr Philippa Kaye

Coping with Diverticulitis
Peter Cartwright

Coping with Dyspraxia
Jill Eckersley

Coping with Early-onset Dementia
Jill Eckersley

**Coping with Eating Disorders
and Body Image**
Christine Craggs-Hinton

Coping with Envy
Dr Windy Dryden

**Coping with Epilepsy in Children
and Young People**
Susan Elliot-Wright

Coping with Family Stress
Dr Peter Cheevers

Coping with Gout
Christine Craggs-Hinton

Coping with Hay Fever
Christine Craggs-Hinton

Coping with Headaches and Migraine
Alison Frith

Coping with Hearing Loss
Christine Craggs-Hinton

Overcoming Common Problems Series

Overcoming Common Problems Series

Living with Osteoporosis
Dr Joan Gomez

Living with Physical Disability and Amputation
Dr Keren Fisher

Living with a Problem Drinker: Your survival guide
Rolande Anderson

Living with Rheumatoid Arthritis
Philippa Pigache

Living with Schizophrenia
Dr Neel Burton and Dr Phil Davison

Living with a Seriously Ill Child
Dr Jan Aldridge

Living with a Stoma
Professor Craig A. White

Living with Tinnitus and Hyperacusis
Dr Laurence McKenna, Dr David Baguley
and Dr Don McFerran

Losing a Child
Linda Hurcombe

Losing a Parent
Fiona Marshall

Menopause in Perspective
Philippa Pigache

Motor Neurone Disease: A family affair
Dr David Oliver

The Multiple Sclerosis Diet Book
Tessa Buckley

Natural Treatments for Arthritis
Christine Craggs-Hinton

Osteoporosis: Prevent and treat
Dr Tom Smith

Overcome Your Fear of Flying
Professor Robert Bor, Dr Carina Eriksen
and Margaret Oakes

Overcoming Agoraphobia
Melissa Murphy

Overcoming Anorexia
Professor J. Hubert Lacey, Christine Craggs-Hinton
and Kate Robinson

Overcoming Depression
Dr Windy Dryden and Sarah Opie

Overcoming Emotional Abuse
Susan Elliot-Wright

Overcoming Gambling: A guide for problem and compulsive gamblers
Philip Mawer

Overcoming Hurt
Dr Windy Dryden

Overcoming Insomnia
Susan Elliot-Wright

Overcoming Jealousy
Dr Windy Dryden

Overcoming Panic and Related Anxiety Disorders
Margaret Hawkins

Overcoming Procrastination
Dr Windy Dryden

Overcoming Shyness and Social Anxiety
Dr Ruth Searle

Overcoming Tiredness and Exhaustion
Fiona Marshall

Reducing Your Risk of Cancer
Dr Terry Priestman

Self-discipline: How to get it and how to keep it
Dr Windy Dryden

The Self-Esteem Journal
Alison Waines

Sinusitis: Steps to healing
Dr Paul Carson

Stammering: Advice for all ages
Renée Byrne and Louise Wright

Stress-related Illness
Dr Tim Cantopher

Ten Steps to Positive Living
Dr Windy Dryden

Therapy for Beginners: How to get the best out of counselling
Professor Robert Bor, Sheila Gill and Anne Stokes

Think Your Way to Happiness
Dr Windy Dryden and Jack Gordon

Tranquillizers and Antidepressants: When to take them, how to stop
Professor Malcolm Lader

The Traveller's Good Health Guide
Dr Ted Lankester

Treating Arthritis Diet Book
Margaret Hills

Treating Arthritis: The drug-free way
Margaret Hills and Christine Horner

Treating Arthritis: More ways to a drug-free life
Margaret Hills

Understanding Obsessions and Compulsions
Dr Frank Tallis

Understanding Traumatic Stress
Dr Nigel Hunt and Dr Sue McHale

When Someone You Love Has Dementia
Susan Elliot-Wright

When Someone You Love Has Depression
Barbara Baker

I dedicate this book to my daughter Christine who has worked with me since the inception of my clinic. As the years go by and my energies wane, she will follow in my footsteps and continue my work of treatment for arthritis sufferers
MH

To John, Joe, Rachel and Jonathan
JH

Contents

Acknowledgements

Grateful thanks are due to Susie Dinan, Assistant Training and Development Officer for London Central YMCA, Research Assistant, University Department of Geriatric Medicine, Royal Free Hospital, Exercise Therapist at St George's Hospitals, Wandsworth Community Trust and holder of the EXA (The National Exercise Association of England) Special Achievement Award, who devised the exercises for this book and whose help and advice were invaluable.

Thanks, also, to Helen Mahood for providing the illustrations.

Introduction

Margaret Hills' own story

On 4 March 1925, I was born two months prematurely. As a four-month-old baby, I suffered 'croup' and developed lock-jaw as a complication of this disease. I was very ill and on two occasions I was given two hours to live, but to everybody's surprise, I survived. My later childhood was similarly beset by ill health and it seemed that I was always sick. I was also underweight, so my mother did everything in her power to nourish me, feeding me on butter, cream, milk, and cheese. My parents had a farm and I was fed on the 'fat of the land'. I feel that this diet, contrary to my parents' good intentions, was largely responsible for me developing arthritis. The high levels of lactic acid it contained were too much for my system to cope with and the result was severe rheumatoid arthritis.

It September 1946, at the age of 21, I started training as a nurse at St Stephen's Hospital, London. I was funloving and carefree, loved to dance, cycle and swim, and my greatest ambition was to be a good nurse. During that first year, things went wonderfully well and I loved my chosen career. Discipline was very strict and the work was hard, but the rewards made it all worth while.

Early in April 1947, I began to feel unwell. I was taken to the nurses' sick bay and the doctor diagnosed acute rheumatoid arthritis. It was also discovered that I had a badly enlarged heart, so I was confined to bed and told to have a period of complete rest, not even being allowed to wash or feed myself. A Harley Street heart specialist was consulted, and he came every other day to examine my heart while the Medical Superintendent noted my progress daily.

At this time, I was suffering severe pain and discomfort. I was

1

being nursed between blankets and, because I could not bear the weight of the bedclothes, I had to cradle to protect my painful limbs. I lay in bed totally helpless for four months, then, gradually, I was allowed to sit out of bed and wash and feed myself. The only treatment I received apart from complete rest was aspirin. In those days, we did not have the vast array of drugs for arthritis that are available today – and, in retrospect, what a blessing that was! In my daily work, treating the sufferers of arthritis at my own clinic, I can see the devastation that can be brought about by the side-effects of the drugs given for arthritis and I thank God that they were not available when I first suffered from it.

. After five months, I was allowed to leave the hospital to go home to convalesce. Before I left, the Medical Superintendent came to see me. He told me that because I had been very ill and my heart had been very badly enlarged, I was never to dance, cycle or swim again. I was not to run uphill or upstairs, and not come back to finish my training as the work was too hard and would put too much strain on my heart. Also, if I ever got married, I was never to have children, and I had to be prepared for recurrences of the disease.

All this was very good advice, and, indeed, faced with the same set of circumstances, I would probably give the same advice to a patient of mine today – the condition of an enlarged heart should not be taken lightly. However, I was young and, looking back, foolish, and I decided to ignore all the advice, to take a chance. I resolved to do what I wanted to do, when I wanted, and I did not tell my parents the advice I had been given. I adopted a 'don't care' attitude and resolved to enjoy any time I had left. I danced, cycled and swam at every opportunity and really threw caution to the wind. At the end of three months, I was quite surprised to find that I was still alive!

Becoming a nurse was still my main objective, so I wrote to the matron of St Stephen's Hospital and asked her if I could resume my training as I was now feeling quite well. I was delighted when she agreed, so back to the hospital I went.

By now, osteoarthritis was beginning to set in and, from time to time, I suffered great pain. However, I managed to get through my training and, on passing my finals, I was given the job of staff nurse in the operating theatre. This was the hardest job in the hospital, but I loved the work and was determined to take each day at a time and live as normal a life as possible. Standing for long hours at the operating table proved to be very painful; my back ached and my legs ached, but I carried on. I had achieved my ambition to be a fully trained nurse and I was so grateful to be given this chance that I wanted to make the most of it.

I met my husband to be at the Hammersmith Palais and we were married the following year. We moved to Coventry and I took a job as an industrial nurse there. My husband wanted a big family and I was determined that he should have one. At that time I do not think that either of us realized how serious the disease I was suffering from was. I remembered being advised not have children, but I took no notice of it, and, each time I became pregnant, I thanked God and prayed that everything would be all right, and it was.

The arthritis got steadily worse, but my panel doctor was most supportive, encouraging me each time by saying, 'you know Mrs Hills, sometimes when a lady has a baby, the acids leave the body'. I lived in hope, but the acids remained. I had six children and we adored them, always doing our best for them, but then I had a recurrence of rheumatoid arthritis that left me completely crippled – every joint was locked tight.

My experience in hospital had made me realize that the medical profession could not cure arthritis and, the more I suffered, the more fearful I became; the future looked bleak. My faith has always been very strong and so, even in my darkest hours, I did not lose hope that one day something would happen to rid me of this dreadful disease.

Through the years, I had researched the cause of the disease – too much uric acid in the body, which comes from the food and drink consumed. The lactic acid that was contained in much of my diet as I grew up – butter, cheese, milk, and cream – had created excess uric acid in my body and this was what was causing all the trouble. I tried many so-called cures, but without success. Then, I worked out the detoxification programme that I dispense to my patients through my clinic now, and it rid me of all signs of arthritis in just 12 months. That was 32 years ago, and I have had a wonderful, pain-free life during those years, though a certain stiffness persisted for a very long time. Gradually, however, because of the various exercises I did, this also disappeared and for years I have had no trouble at all.

What a joy life became when my arthritis disappeared. I devoted my life to bringing up our children because just being able to bath them, wash their hair, cook their meals, collect them from school – every mundane job – was precious to me. I had two more children when I regained my health, eight in all. They are all healthy, intelligent, well-balanced human beings and for this I give thanks daily. For 30 years I did not go out to work, just concentrated on home life, and loved every minute of it, but all good things come to an end. One by one the children got married and soon the nest was empty apart from my husband and myself. I then had too much time on my hands, so I decided to pick up my career as a nurse.

I took a refresher course in nursing at our local hospital, and started working for an agency as a district nurse, as well as helping out in factory surgeries. I soon got back into the routine of working and I did enjoy it, except when I had to give injections from time to time to sufferers of arthritis. I did not like doing this because I knew that the side-effects could be most damaging.

I worked for the agency for six years and then, on 19 June 1982, an article appeared in the *Coventry Evening Telegraph*. It read as follows: 'Nobody knows what causes arthritis. There is no cure for it. The Coventry Council are spending ['x'] amounts of money on research and in three years, they hope to come up with a cure.' Needless to say, to date, they still have not found a cure and, in my opinion, never will while they look to drugs to provide the answer. When I read this article, I felt compelled to pick up my pen and write to the paper, telling them of my experience in getting rid of my own arthritis. When they received my letter, they telephoned me to ask for my photograph. I reluctantly

4

agreed and they printed my story. Then the dilemma began.

My telephone never stopped ringing; as soon as I answered one call, there was another sufferer of arthritis on the line. I had to take the phone off the hook to get any peace and I was finding it hard to do my work. During the two remaining weeks in June, over 4000 letters cascaded through my letter-box. Eventually, the postman asked if he could leave them in bundles on the doorstep. I had treatment leaflets printed and sent one to each person who wrote and, between June and September, I sent treatment leaflets to people in practically every country in the world. I gave up my work with the agency and made appointments at my home, charging $5 a time to help cover printing costs and any mone left over I gave to charity. Thus my clinic began.

I soon realized that the number of people suffering from arthritis was great and I could not hope to reach enough people on a one-to-one basis at the clinic, so I started to book hotel rooms at weekends, giving talks and advising people this way. It was not unusual to have 300 to 400 people turn up to the talks, and at one talk I gave in Ireland, over 900 people came and several hundred had to be turned away for lack of room. Sometimes the numbers waiting to hear the talks were so great that as soon as I finished one talk, I had to start another.

A typical example of the press reports made following the talks is this one:

Phone Calls Galore Over Arthritis Talk

Arthritis sufferers searching for a cure besieged a hotel near Stourbridge which staged a talk on natural methods of healing this painful condition. Now the nurse who gave the talk has appealed for people to get in touch with her instead of bombarding the Stewponey Hotel at Stourton with phone calls. More than two hundred people turned up at the talk given by Nurse Margaret Hills on Saturday and an extra session had to be put on for dozens of others who had to be turned away. The hotel manager said, 'The response has been unbelievable – the phone has not stopped ringing. I never realised that there was so much concern about arthritis. We must have had more than 1000 phone calls since the talk was reported.'

All this made me realize that the amount of suffering is astronomical. Furthermore, the disease affects so many people in every country of the world. It was this realization that resulted in my decision to send out details of my system of treatment by post, which applied to all people with arthritis as the symptoms are much the same for all; it is just that the effects are suffered to a greater or lesser degree. The system works extremely well, and we liaise with the parents' doctors when necessary. Most doctors are very helpful, and when they see the improvement in their patients, they become very interested.

In 1985, I wrote my first book, *Treating Arthritis: The drug-free way* (Sheldon Press). Through this, the Margaret Hills Clinic has become known throughout the world. Patients from many countries come for appointments and those who cannot come are sent details of the treatment by post.

My daughter, Christine, has been with me at the clinic from the beginning. Through the years, she has learned my methods of treatment and has carried out extensive studies into the alternative, holistic way of treating arthritis and, as a result of these studies and experience, has become well versed in the medical side. She has now attained the professional qualification of ECNP – European Certified Nutritional Practitioner. We have engaged various other members of staff to help guide people with their treatment. The results of all our work are very gratifying, and the following letters will give you an idea of the success we have had.

The following is an extract from a letter sent to me by Mr and Mrs E. It tells of their 14-year-old daughter, who suffered from very severe juvenile arthritis. I treated her for nearly two years.

My wife and I are both over the moon with the progress that Fiona has made and so is the paediatrician, Dr S. He discharged her from outpatients on her last visit. He was amazed at her progress and commented that whatever you are treating her with, it is doing nothing but good and should have all the credit. I shudder to think what would have been the outcome if we had kept her on the drugs.

The 'before and after' photographs I have of this girl show remarkable differences in her health.

Another amazing story is that of Mrs N. I treated this lady for 18 months for very severe osteoarthritis. Her hands were quite badly deformed and swollen. The following is an extract from a letter she wrote to me on 9 December 1993.

Dear Mrs Hills,
I had an appointment at the hospital to see the Orthopaedic Surgeon on October 28th. He discussed my treatment with you. He had me walking to him to see how I walked and then he examined my knees. He was amazed at the improvement and said something was working. He asked me to stay on your treatment for a further six months, when he would take more X-rays.

This lady's hands are no longer deformed or swollen, and, here again, the photos I have of her before and after treatment have to be seen to be believed, so dramatic is the improvement.

I discharged Mrs C. on 23 January 1994 and she wrote me the following letter a short while afterwards.

Having visited your clinic for the last time, I felt I must write and thank you for your help and kindness during the past few years. To be rid of arthritis and the pain it brings is a marvellous feeling and I can't tell you how thankful I am that I bought your book *Treating Arthritis: The drug-free way*. Having had arthritis in almost every moveable joint in my body and to be free of pain is almost unbelievable and not a drug in sight. Once again, many many thanks and long may you continue to help arthritis sufferers.

The following letter came from Mrs M.

Dear Nurse Hills,
Thank you for writing your book *Treating Arthritis: The drug-free way* and for making your treatment available. Over nine months as a postal patient. I have regained full use of my right hand and am now free from constant pain.

Mrs Childs of Rugby sent me the following letter.

To whom this may concern,
I am writing this letter just to say that I suffered with rheumatoid arthritis for nearly two years. It started after being away on holiday in Cyprus. When I came back, one of my knees had doubled in size and I was getting horrific pains in my legs – I used to cry with pain.

My doctor sent me to see a specialist at the hospital, as by then it had moved to my wrists and I did not know what to do because of all the pain I was getting. I could not even write a note for my daughter for school because it looked as if a five-year-old had written it. I was given painkillers and even then I was still in pain. I was given splints to sleep in at night, also splints for the day. I honestly thought I would be like this for the rest of my life, until a friend of my husband bought me your book – *Treating Arthritis: The drug-free way*. I have taken all the advice it contained and now I have been discharged from the hospital and suffer no pain at all. I'm just writing this in the hope that it will give someone somewhere faith in what you say. Thank you Margaret Hills SRN.

Letters such as these arrive on my desk daily and I could continue to give case history after case history of patients who have benefitted from our treatment, if space would allow. Suffice it to say, though, that all types of arthritis can be treated if my plan is carried out as advised.

The types of arthritis

The main types of arthritis are *juvenile arthritis* (rheumatoid arthritis in children), *adult rheumatoid arthritis, osteoarthritis* and *psoriatic arthritis*. Let us look at these more closely.

Juvenile arthritis

Quite a number of children who suffer from arthritis come to my clinic. Unfortunately, arthritis can be inherited and the pain and stiffness it produces in children is very sad to see. It affects the coverings of the bones of the joints simultaneously or successively, making every movement agony, and life becomes dull, boring, and painful. Sports activities and schoolwork suffer. Parents don't know what to do to rectify the situation, so they call in the doctor. Blood tests and X-rays conform that the child has rheumatoid arthritis. Bed rest in hospital may follow, where the child may be put into traction and given drugs to treat the arthritis – sometimes non-steroidal drugs, such as Brufen, Indocid, Feldene and so on, sometimes steroids. The drugs work for a little while and the patient, who feels better, is allowed to go home, but, unfortunately, the improvement is short-lived. The effects of the drugs wear off and the pain and stiffness return with full force. As drugs and pain can drain the body of iron, the patient may become anaemic. The doctor is called again, the dosage of the drug is increased or a stronger drug is given and the story repeats itself. It is a very sad situation for the parents as well as the child – they are virtually powerless to help when their child cries with pain day and night. Nobody gets any sleep and the resulting tension and frustration can cause real problems in the family. Very often, too, the child has gained so much weight as a side-effect of the drugs or because of inactivity due to the pain of the illness, that it takes both parents to lift them out of bed just to go to the toilet.

Rheumatoid arthritis in children is very serious as, quite frequently, it causes inflammation of the membrane lining the heart valves, which, in many cases, leads to permanent heart damage.

One theory about the cause of rheumatoid arthritis is that it is due primarily to infection by *Streptococcus* bacteria, but for the *Streptococcus* to survive and produce the disease, there must also be secondary causal factors. Enlarged tonsils and adenoids are important predisposing factors. The cold, wet, changes of temperature, and fatigue may also act as predisposing factors.

A sore throat, irregular joint pains, and a slight malaise may arise as preliminary symptoms, but, as a rule, the onset is abrupt and the disease is fully established within 24 hours. Then, the joints are swollen and painful, the face is flushed, there are profuse sweats, the throat is often sore, the temperature high, and the pain causes sleeplessness. There is also loss of appetite, thirst, constipation, and hightly coloured urine. The knees, wrists, elbows, and shoulders are red, hot, tender, and extremely painful on movement. Inflammation wanders from joint to joint, from day to day – one joint recovering as another is attacked. In uncomplicated cases, the acute symptoms subside within about ten days, but relapses are very common.

Arthritis in adults

Rheumatoid arthritis

Rheumatoid arthritis is a very serious disease. It is much more common in children and young adults than it is in older people, and it is much more common in women than men.

All the symptoms mentioned under Juvenile arthritis above are experienced by adults. The disease usually begins with a flu-like condition, which invariably includes a sore throat. The joints feel hot and painful, there is a high temperature and sometimes a rash, very often down the fronts of the legs. The heart, too, can become involved as inflammation of the muscle of the heart is common and, of course, this can be very serious.

Every joint in the body becomes affected and, in severe cases, there is widespread destruction of soft tissue as well, including the skin, heart, lungs, liver and kidneys. The majority of sufferers experience pain in practically every joint – the knuckles, wrists, elbows, hips, spine, knees, ankles and feet, and the neck and shoulders, too.

In my opinion, and as stated earlier and in my first book (*Treating Arthritis: The drug-free way*, Sheldon Press, 1985), the root cause of the problem is uric acid in the body. Uric acid is a wonderful source of food for *Streptococcus* bacteria. When the body is attacked by this virus, first there is a sore throat, then the virus gets into the bloodstream, causing severe pain and discomfort in the body. Very often there is a high temperature, which is the result of the immune system trying to fight it off. If the patient has a body full of toxic acids, which have arisen as a result of bad eating habits, smoking, drinking and so on, the immune system is weak and the *Streptococcus* takes over, creating havoc within the patient's body. Equally, if the body is cleansed of toxic acids, the virus cannot live because the immune system is strong and can protect the body; the patient is none the worse for the attack.

When the patient becomes victim to rheumatoid arthritis, there is only one sensible course of action – to remove the toxic acids from the body. Through the years, and particularly since I opened the Margaret Hills Clinic for Arthritis, I have treated many thousands of patients and my experience has been that a detoxification programme to eliminate the toxic acids, in conjunction with a specific nutritional regime, works wonders in relieving rheumatoid and osteoarthritis, as well as polymyalgia rheumatica, which, in my opinion, is caused by toxic acids in the muscles.

High quality nutrition, therefore, is very important, and, because I have realized that the majority of the public do not recognize good-quality vitamin and mineral supplements in the shops, I have produced a complete nutritional supplement of my own that is showing excellent results. It is called Margaret Hills' Formula for Arthritics. Protein, too, is a must, because arthritis is a disease that weakens the muscles and protein helps with muscle strength (providing there is not a porteinurea condition). This I have also had made in a supplement form that is specially suitable for sufferers of arthritis. It contains phenylalanine, which is an excellent natural pain blocker.

The thyroid gland becomes very involved in both rheumatoid and osteoarthritis. If one of my patients has not had a thyroid test, I send a note to their doctor requesting one. I also request a test for anaemia, which so many people with arthritis suffer from. Doctors are very co-operative in this respect.

Prevention of osteoporosis is very important for anyone with arthritis and so taking a good calcium supplement is a must. Note, though, that this mineral should never be taken without the inclusion of vitamin D as this vitamin enables the body to absorb the calcium. The Margaret Hills Formula for Arthritics includes this important mineral.

A large number of elderly patients who visit the clinic have been prescribed hormone replacement therapy in order to combat osteoporosis, but this is a constant source of worry to me. This therapy, prescribed so freely, is not the answer as it very often upsets the nutritional balance in the body, especially that of zinc, which is so very important for the immune system. Levels of magnesium and vitamin B6, too, can be affected. If you want to know more about this, I suggest you read an interesting book by Dr Ellen Grant, *Sexual Chemistry*. In it she states that prescribed hormones are, in her opinion, behind the dramatic increases there have been in the incidence of breast, early cervical, ovarian, and endometrial cancer that we are seeing so much of now.

Osteoarthritis

Osteoarthritis often starts with pain in a particular joint, such as in a finger. It is the most common disorder of the joints and is estimated to be present in 80 to 90 per cent of people over the age of 60. The condition is more common in women that in men. Osteoarthritis is characterized by the gradual destruction of the central parts of the cartilage lining the affected joints, while, at the same time, there is overgrowth of the outer part of the cartilage, which, ultimately, results in the growth of bony spurs. It is very often accompanied by obesity, which results in stresses and strains being put on the weight-bearing joints, namely the lower spine, hips, knees, ankles, and feet. The shoulder joints can also suffer, however. In chronic cases, the joint becomes enlarged and deformed. There is seldom any generalized disturbance to the well-being of the sufferer, such as fever or malaise. The diagnosis is confirmed by an X-ray examination.

Hip and knee replacements are not uncommon treatments in cases where the disease has become quite severe. Otherwise, treatment consists of very gentle exercise and sparing the joints. Local heat and spa baths are particularly helpful. Indeed, according to a French study, spa therapy can produce long-lasting improvements in lower back pain (it has a similar effect in cases of rheumatoid arthritis). The study was of 104 patients who had had lower back pain for at least two years. They received a underwater spa treatment over three weeks. Immediately after the treatment, patients showed significant reductions in the duration and severity of pain they experienced and, nine months later, this improvement had remained with them. Their use of analgesics fell by almost 60 per cent.

Psoriatic arthritis

In my opinion, the reason for psoriasis is the underlying general toxic condition of the body.

Many of my patients suffer dreadfully as a result of this condition. They first make an appointment because of their arthritis, not realizing that the arthritis and psoriasis are connected. As the arthritis clears as a result of following the diet and treatment we prescribe for them, the psoriasis lessens and eventually disappears.

The psoriasis almost always appears first around the backs of the elbows and fronts of the knees. Patches also appear on other parts of the body – the scalp and face especially – and sometimes it invades the whole body.

Just like arthritis, there is no *medical* cure for the condition, but, speaking from my experience and the remarkable results we get at my clinic, all this is needed is a complete detoxification programme and attention to general health. Results do not happen overnight – it takes daily commitment from the patient for the required amount of time.

Exercise and arthritis

Very often, during the course of my work, people ask about

exercise. So far, I have had to advise them one by one, but now, I am very excited about the publication of this book as I know that this tremendous source of help will be available to all those who need it. The human body is designed for activity – all bodily functions degenerate and atrophy without use – so it is very important that we all exercise properly, but it is especially important for the sufferers of arthritis to do so. I wish you well in all your efforts to help yourself to health.

1

What Exercise Can Do For You

We cannot fail to be aware of the benefits of regular physical activity and, certainly, people who make an exercise routine an integral part of their lives do seem to have more energy to cope with the demands of daily life. Their hearts, lungs, and muscles work efficiently, so they have more stamina. Also, regular, controlled programmes produce stronger muscles and bones, supple joints, good co-ordination and balance, which help them to do more without straining.

People who exercise regularly often look better too. Their complexion is clear and glowing, their hair shines, they have good posture and appear confident. All these can be the benefits of a good programme of enjoyable activity.

Of course, other important elements in life play a part, too. Eating a well-balanced diet, which includes plenty of fresh, unprocessed foods and a good supply of the essential vitamins and minerals, enjoying the company of family and friends, using activity and relaxation to relieve any stress, sleeping better, being less prone to infection and illness all link together and help to make us fully healthy.

If you have arthritis, the idea that regular physical activity can improve your condition may seem out of the question. Even if you have led an active life until recently, you will now be tempted to stop, feeling that limited mobility and pain put you, literally, out of the running. This is not the case. If you have osteoarthritis, regular exercise will *not* wear your joints out and make your condition worse. On the contrary, by moving more, you will increase joint protection by stimulating the production of synovial fluid, which coats the ends of the joints and is absorbed by the spongy cartilage. Like oil, this thick substance lubricates your joints and may help to prevent further damage. Lack of synovial fluid reduces protection of the joints and can also contribute to the pain of osteoarthritis.

If you already take part in regular physical activity, you may need to adapt what you do. To reduce the risk of damage, it is recommended that you swap playing contact sports, such as rugby and 'explosive' games, such as squash, for activities that put less strain on the joints.

With all forms of arthritis, it is important to combine exercise with rest and to do a few carefully controlled simple mobility and stretching movements once or twice a day, even when the joints are swollen and painful. With rheumatoid or other inflammatory types of arthritis, you need to keep a delicate balance between activity and rest so that you can take advantage of the times when your arthritis is in remission to put your joints through their full range of movement and build up muscle strength so that you can help prevent stiffening or deformity of the joints.

If your arthritis affects your back and spine, as in ankylosing spondylitis, you will need to keep as mobile as possible.

For all types of arthritis, gently moving the joints and stretching the muscles and tendons is the best way to relieve strain on painful joints, improve body alignment, and help you feel more relaxed and in control of your disease.

Of course, rest is important, too, particularly during acute phases, as it can help to lessen the inflammation, but too much inactivity makes the condition worse. Experts now advise you to exercise as much as you can to increase movement, strength, improve the functioning of the joints, and create better all-round physical well-being.

But you need to keep a balance. Adjust the amount of rest and exercise according to the stage of your disease and how you feel each day. Too much exercise will put you at risk of exhaustion, injury, and more pain. Just be aware of the temptation to do too much. Learn to listen to your body and know when it is telling you to take things easy.

Ideally, you should aim to do some movements every day. In Chapter 3, you will see that we have chosen exercises that, when put together, form an easy programme that can be carried out each day in just a few minutes. Once you begin to know the different movements (this will only take a few days), these particular exercises can easily become part of your daily life – a good habit, like brushing your teeth, something you know you have to do every day.

The four areas

To exercise successfully and safely, and to benefit fully from this, you need to work on four areas: flexibility, muscle strength, motor fitness and stamina. All four contribute to your overall fitness. This is why some apparently sporty people may not be as fully fit as they appear. Weightlifters may seem strong, but they are doing little for their circulation and even less for their flexibility – the most important area to work on if you have arthritis of any kind.

Flexibility

If your muscles are flexible, you can move easily. Flexibility is reduced by your muscles tightening and shortening as this limits your range of movement. Put simply, if you do not use it, you lose it. Many adults lose their suppleness through sheer lack of activity, but they manage to get through daily life because there is no specific pain or injury. However, they are always at risk of an unexpected strain or sprain because of this stiffness.

If you have arthritis, there may be pain in one or more joints and you may hesitate to move too much in case this increases the pain. The less you move your muscles, however, the stiffer your joints become, and the greater the likelihood of increased pain.

If your arthritis is very mild, or just in the early stages, keeping supple may well be a simple matter of maintenance. Each day you need to take your joints through their full natural range of movement so that you can reach, bend, stretch, and turn without strain. The exercises in Chapter 3 will show you exactly how to do this safely.

If your arthritis is more severe and disabling, working on your flexibility, using slow, gentle movements, will keep your joints lubricated and prevent further deformation. Some passive, mobilizing exercises can be done on bad days, using a pole or hoop to prevent the joint moving too much. Alternatively, a qualified physiotherapist can help ease your joints into movement for you.

For sufferers of ankylosing spondylitis, regular back mobility and flexibility exercises are vital as they will help keep the affected areas as mobile as possible.

Suppleness makes a tremendous difference to everyday life if you have arthritis. It can mean the difference between dependence and independence. Dressing, putting on shoes or stockings, reaching up to a shelf, climbing stairs or getting in and out of a car, can be so much easier when your joints are more flexible, and you run far less risk of injury, too.

Muscle strength and endurance

This is vital for good posture and helps us put less strain on the joints. Muscles and tendons help ligaments to support the joints when they move, and protect them from injury. The stronger your muscles, the more stable your joints will be. If you have strong back, buttock, and abdominal muscles, your posture will improve – you will stand straight with less effort, and your joints will be taking less of the strain.

If you have pain, your natural reaction is to move the affected joint less. Rest is essential from time to time, and it may not be possible to do strengthening exercises on bad days, but even the smallest movement will help prevent muscles and tendons from shortening and weakening. A balance between rest and exercise is needed to allow you to retain muscle strength and length without putting the painful joint under too much weight-bearing pressure.

Muscle *strength* will enable you to move and lift quite heavy weights efficiently and safely. Muscle *endurance* gives you the staying power you need to complete quite simple tasks, such as carrying bags of shopping or beating a cake mixture, without becoming exhausted. It takes time to gain strength and endurance, but these can be built up slowly and safely by gentle repetitive movements. These need to be done regularly if you are not to lose this level of strength and endurance.

If you are one of the unfortunate few who suffer from osteoporosis *and* arthritis, you need to be extra cautious. Osteoporosis is a decrease in bone density, which increases the risk of fractures. Regular load-bearing exercises, done carefully, are essential for you. These include brisk walking, back strengthening and squeezing tennis balls in your hands.

Motor fitness

This is a vital area as this kind of fitness helps you to control your movements. Through it you can improve your skills of balance, co-ordination, and your ability to react speedily. As you get older, this is a part of general fitness that can be forgotten, and it is all the more important to work on it if you have arthritis.

When you have pain, particularly in the hips, knees or feet, this naturally affects how you stand (your posture), the way you walk, and balance. You may be afraid of tripping or stumbling, especially if the pain makes it hard to lift your feet or bend your knees. Exercises to improve your balance will help to make you feel a lot more secure.

Stamina

Stamina means you have the energy to keep going. The pain and distress of arthritis can be debilitating and tiring, so by building up physical stamina, you give yourself an extra boost. Your stamina is largely dependent on a healthy cardiovascular system – the heart and blood vessels – and respiratory system – the lungs. Their job is to transport oxygen from the lungs to the muscles and organs, and the more efficiently they do this, the more energy you have.

The word 'aerobic' is used to describe the system that carries oxygen from the air to the muscles and 'aerobic exercise' is any form of exercise that helps improve the functioning of this system. Oxygen is transported from the lungs in the bloodstream to the body and the working muscles. Regular exercise results in a heart that pumps efficiently which means it can respond quickly as soon as extra oxygen is needed. The muscles then use the oxygen, together with the fuel derived from food, to produce a steady amount of energy.

Aerobic exercise is the only way to improve stamina, but you do not have to wear a leotard or jogging suit and risk jarring your joints on a hard floor in order to achieve results! You can improve your cardio-respiratory system by doing any form of sustained exercise that makes you slightly breathless. Your muscles should also feel a little tired. You will feel this way after walking briskly for a while, cycling, whether outdoors or on an exercise bike, while swimming or doing water exercises.

Initially, three to four minutes of continuous (that is, without any breaks!) aerobic exercise is quite sufficient. The length of time can be increased gradually over the weeks. Most experts recommend building up to a 20-minute session of sustained aerobic exercise 3 to 4 times a week as a way of gaining aerobic fitness, and then 2 to 3 sessions a week to sustain it. As you build up to a full-length session, you can check your progress by using the 'talk test'. While you do your chosen activity you should feel you are working hard – your breathing will be heavier, your heart will beat faster, you will feel warm – but you should be able to hold a normal conversation (count or recite a poem to yourself) without being out of breath. If you are completely breathless, then you are doing too much.

Always warm up before exercising and have a cooling down session afterwards. This gives the muscles a chance to adapt to the demands made on them. Remembering to breathe deeply and evenly throughout the session also helps.

A bonus of stamina-building exercise is that it burns off calories and uses body fat as energy. Provided you do not compensate for extra activity by eating more or drinking alcohol or sugary drinks afterwards to quench your thirst, you will gradually lose any extra weight, which might be putting strain on your arthritic joints.

Another benefit of regular physical activity is that it will make it easier to give up the bad habits that affect your health, such as smoking and drinking too much alcohol. You will also sleep better and find you depend less on drugs to deal with headaches. All the evidence shows that people who do aerobic exercise regularly are less at risk of heart attacks and strokes than people who do not.

By exercising these four areas of fitness, you will give yourself a chance to gain (or regain) a level of physical fitness that will be of tremendous benefit. You will be fit for life. You may not become an Olympic athlete or a world champion, and exercise on its own can never be a cure for arthritis, but your body was designed to move and, by making the decision to keep it moving, you will give it the vital extra support it needs to cope with the disease.

2

Exercise Can Help You Feel Better

The trouble with chronic disease like arthritis is that you may often have had the feeling that there is very little you can do to change things. You listen to the advice of experts such as doctors and consultants who tell you that your arthritis is unlikely to go away. You hear friends and family telling you simply to come to terms with the disease and adapt your life accordingly. This can make you feel quite helpless and depressed. Your life seems to be ruled by your arthritis and you can feel that there is little that you can do about it.

You may also feel angry or bitter when you are told you have a chronic illness. You can feel robbed of all sorts of things – the freedom to do what you want, when you want to without pain, the loss of the life you have led so far. There may be resentment. If you are young you may feel that you are being cheated as you see others of your own age leading apparently full, active lives. If you are older, you may dislike being told that this is to be expected at your age. Whatever messages you receive, they may be very negative and will encourage you to see a bleak future for yourself. Often those who are trying to be kind and helpful may just reinforce your sense of helplessness and not allow you to be positive.

All these feelings are understandable, and it is good to recognise them rather than ignore them. If you feel very depressed or uncomfortable about your anger and sadness, you may find it helpful to see a counsellor and talk things through. They can help you to see things more clearly and regain your self-esteem, a sense of pride in yourself and what you are achieving now and what you can achieve in the future. Yet, you may also want to rebel against this, not want to accept it, and want to fight it.

Exercise can help here as the physical benefits will spill over and benefit your emotional health. The body influences the mind and vice versa. Regular exercise of any kind will not only enhance your physical fitness, it can also help you feel a great deal more positive about yourself and your life. You will begin to feel calmer, more confident in your abilities to cope. You will sense that you have gained inner strength. If you follow a safe series of movements and know that each move you make is actually going to help your joints to function better and lessen some of the pain, this can give a tremendous boost to your determination not to let the disease get the better of you. Also, exercise, even at quite an elementary level, as well as making you physically fitter, can really help you to feel a great deal more positive about yourself and your condition. This is because, when you make the decision to exercise, you are actively doing something for yourself that will help your arthritis.

When we are ill we tend to wait for others to lead the way. You take the drugs prescribed for your arthritis, but are not really fully involved in the decision to do so; the doctor prescribes the drugs, you take them. However, each time you exercise, you make a positive choice to use your body, move it, improve it. Initially you may receive help from a physiotherapist who will show you the sort of movements you can make. If your arthritis is very acute or well advanced, the physiotherapist may be very involved with these movements, sometimes moving the joints for you. This will give you confidence. After this, though, the responsibility is yours to do those movements regularly, maybe two or three times a day. When you do so, you are making the statement that you are not prepared to lie down and let your arthritis walk all over you, that you will do what you can to help yourself.

Of course, there will be times when it is hard to think so positively, when the disease flares up and you are in pain. This is when rest and movement are essential. However, even at these times you can practise listening to your body, sensing what it needs and making your own decision to rest or to do very simple movements rather than a full routine. Decisions like these take you a step nearer to managing your arthritis effectively. *You* are in control, *you* are making the decisions.

23

Most people who exercise regularly talk about the feeling of elation and achievement they have as a result. Often, after a successful session, you will have extra energy. Each time you notice that you have achieved just a little more, have stretched a bit further or been able to do more repetitions of a movement than before, this will boost your self-esteem, you will feel good about yourself.

Handling pain

The one thing that may make you hesitate about starting any exercise is worry about pain. Pain is important – it tells you when you are doing too much and you will probably have already learned ways in which to lead your life that reduce this risk. For example, you will avoid carrying heavy loads, putting pressure on sore joints, you will rest more and so on.

It is worth remembering that there are two types of pain. First, there is sudden, acute pain. This kind of pain tells us we have done some damage and need to do something quickly to relieve it. If this happens during exercise you must stop. Second, there is the chronic pain that goes with most forms of arthritis. During a flare-up, the pain will sharpen, but the rest of the time it will simmer along and colour your days and nights. Even during these times there will be differences. For some of you there may be days when there is little or no pain, while for others, the pain will be there most of the time, making its presence felt.

Of course, pain is a very individual matter – we all have different pain thresholds. What will be sufficiently painful for one person to make them hesitate before doing anything at all, someone else may be fortunate enough to be able to continue with ease. This said, pain is still a warning sign, so you must always take notice of it. There will be times when it is severe and you will need to rest. At other times, exercising gently, without straining, can actually relieve your pain.

Exercise can help pain in three ways. First, remember that if you keep your joints moving, you encourage synovial fluid to flow in and lubricate them. Second, apart from the relaxation they bring, the rhythmic movements of exercise trigger the release of the body's pain-relieving hormones, endorphins. Third, when you exercise, you begin to feel relaxed and this can help break the vicious circle of pain, tension, and depression in which many people with arthritis become trapped. This occurs because, when you are in pain, your body naturally tenses up as a reaction to discomfort. This tension makes the pain worse, so you tense up more. At the same time, the pain can depress you and the depression can lead to further tension, causing further pain.

It is natural to worry that exercise may cause more pain if you have arthritis. This can be a psychological barrier for you to leap, especially if you have been inactive and walking on egg shells for some time. You need to have sufficient confidence to trust your body, to know that if you learn to move it in the right way, you will not cause *more* pain, but *less*. You may find that you gain this reassurance from an expert, such as a qualified physiotherapist or qualified exercise teacher. They will show you which movements to do and correct you while you do them. They will be able to help you learn which exercises to choose and how to make slight adjustments to your position until you gain maximum benefit from them. If supervised exercise is not possible, then the very gentle exercises in Chapter 3 will allow you to progress and adapt to moving again in a similar way – very safely, slowly, and carefully. Each time you exercise and experience no pain, you will increase your confidence. As this happens, you will feel relaxed and at ease with your body, which will reduce the likelihood of pain.

When you finish exercising, your body may feel tired, especially in the early stages – this is discomfort, not pain. If there is pain in the joints and it lasts for more than two hours after you have been exercising, then you are probably doing too much and need either to rest or exercise less energetically. If there is stiffness in the muscles the following day, you have definitely exercised too hard for your level of fitness. You could also consider other ways of dealing with your pain so that it does not dominate your life. Relaxation is a very effective way of controlling pain if you remember that tension and anxiety often make you more susceptible to pain. Relaxation techniques, therefore, should become as much part of your life as the more active exercise movements. They are an ideal way to finish an exercise session, but they can also be done at any other time during the day – maybe before you go to sleep or if you wake up in the middle of the night (see Chapter 3 for relaxation routines).

Some people find that visualization techniques help them to deal with pain. You could try something simple, such as thinking of your pain as an enemy trying to conquer your body and imaging an army of pain-relieving cells fighting to overcome it. Alternatively, you could use a gentler image of support and comfort that will soothe the pain in the way you might hold and cuddle a child who is hurt or unwell.

The role of stress

Stress plays an important role in arthritis. There is more and more evidence to show that certain types of arthritis, such as rheumatoid arthritis, are made worse or are even triggered by stress, while the changes produced in the joints that lead to deterioration and osteoarthritis may also be linked to stress. Stress affects arthritis both physically and psychologically. Physically, if you are anxious and worried a lot of the time, then your muscles will be in an almost constant state of tension, making movement of the joints even more difficult. This is because tension restricts blood flow and the supply of oxygen and nutrients to the body. This causes a build-up of lactic acids, which, in turn, causes fatigue and exhaustion.

If your worrying also prevents you from having a restful, uninterrupted night's sleep, it gives your painful joints very little chance to rest and relax. It is natural to worry about your arthritis in the early stages – you may not know how it will affect your life, and, if you have been healthy until now, being unwell comes as a shock. If you have rheumatoid arthritis, you may not know how long it will last, whether it will go into remission, whether there will be further flare-ups.

EXERCISE CAN HELP YOU FEEL BETTER

Our bodies are well equipped to deal with sudden, short-term stress, giving us the extra energy and strength we need to avoid or escape danger. When this happens, our blood pressure rises and the heart pumps more blood quickly to the muscles to prepare for action. When the danger is past, everything settles down to normal, but, if we have long-term stress, this return to normal does not take place. The result is often exhaustion, permanent tiredness and fatigue.

Exercise is one good way in which we can relieve stress. The sense of achievement and the boost to our self-esteem that result are very helpful. Also, as we have seen, the very act of moving around helps you to relax. In turn, this will help you to sleep better, which should help reduce pain, as a peaceful night's sleep gives the muscles and tendons round your painful joints a chance to rest.

The benefits of exercise classes

As well as the regular routines that you will do at home to keep supple and mobile and strengthen your muscles, you may also enjoy going to an exercise class or taking up some activity that involves meeting other people.

At first, you may hesitate, especially if you find movement difficult, but most classes these days are non-competitive. The aim is for everyone to do the best they can without straining. No one has anything to prove to anyone else, and the support you will receive from others will be very helpful and encouraging.

Illness is often isolating and if you have arthritis, it may have meant losing touch with people. Maybe you have had to stop work or go out less because you haven't been well enough. Sharing your exercise with others can create a new social life for you and you will enjoy that special feeling that comes when a group works together.

Initially you may feel happier exercising with other people who also have arthritis. It is good to share experiences and progress, and you can give each other confidence and a feeling of security. As your mobility increases, however, you may also want to join a more general class, perhaps at your local leisure centre.

Sharing your commitment to exercise with others, as well as being an excellent way to make lasting friendships, can help you not to give up, or miss sessions, without a very good reason. There is often an unspoken contract, and a shared determination to keep going. If you have never been to an exercise class before, the sense of caring, laughter, fun and friendship that can be found is something that you need now and can benefit from.

3

Exercise, Rest and Relaxation

First things first

Before starting any exercise routine, please check with your doctor, consultant or physiotherapist that you are in good health and that the movements you plan to do are right for you.

If you feel any of the following, *stop* exercising and seek the advice of your doctor before continuing:

- numbness
- tingling
- dizziness
- nausea
- excessive breathlessness
- pains in the chest, back, neck, face or arms
- pains in the joints.

Remember

If you have arthritis of any kind, you must be careful to ensure that the risks of exercise do not outweigh the benefits. This means that the type of exercise, the amount, frequency, intensity, and the way you do it *must* be right for you – your body, fitness level, type and stage of arthritis. It must also be combined with a period of rest afterwards to ensure maximum benefits. You may need to adjust what you do every day, but the key is to listen to your body rather than your mind. Therefore, avoid exercising a joint when it is painful, especially if you have an inflammatory type of arthritis, such as rheumatoid arthritis. In this case, it is best to rest the joint until the inflammation has reduced.

Before you start

The exercises you are about to do can quite easily be made part of your daily life. If you can do this, then you will give yourself a much better chance of managing your arthritis as well as possible and relieving the pain.

No one pretends that it is easy to exercise regularly – all sorts of things come along to make this tricky – but as more and more people have shown, it can be done. It helps to be aware of the traps before you start.

Overenthusiasm is often more of a hindrance than a help. If you are too enthusiastic at the beginning, you may be tempted to do more exercise than you should. You may then have pain and be forced to stop. So, the rule is to take things nice and slowly, build up gradually, and then the chances of injury are reduced.

If you have arthritis, you will naturally be worried about the pain exercise might cause. You need to understand that if you feel pain while you are exercising or if you have pain after exercise that lasts longer than two hours, you are overexerting yourself and your body will not benefit. Remember pain is a warning sign.

At the same time, you will begin to be able to sense the difference between *pain*, when damage could be done, and *discomfort*, which is usually a sign, particularly in the early days, that you are doing movements that you haven't done for a long time. This is why, for each exercise, we tell you where you should feel the work as your muscles respond. Some exercises may initially be very uncomfortable for you. If this is the case, do not persist, but choose an alternative until you are ready to try again.

To avoid unnecessary pain or discomfort, you should prepare carefully before exercising. Here are some suggestions.

- It is probably best not to exercise immediately after you get up. This is when you are likely to be stiff. If you are a morning person or if your life is such that the morning is the only time when you can do your routines, then you need to get up a little earlier, maybe have a warm bath and move around to help the blood to start flowing before you do your routines. Warmth is essential if you have arthritis, so exercise in a warm, comfortable room, and wear extra layers, such as socks, gloves, a scarf. If you are going to exercise outside, warm up for 20 minutes indoors first.

- Make sure you have a mat or folded blanket if you plan to do any floor exercises.
- If you are to get the most out of the session, you need to be uninterrupted for 15 to 30 minutes, so be firm with the people you live with so that they do not call you to the telephone or front door. If you are on your own, you will have to try to ignore all interruptions. Your exercises are the most important part of your day, so they should have priority.
- Do not exercise immediately after a meal. Allow two hours to digest a light meal and longer if you have eaten meat. If you are taking pain-relieving pills for your arthritis, it is very important not to use them to dull any pain so that you can exercise.

Assessing your fitness level and how your arthritis affects you

Before you start, you also need to know how fit you are and how your arthritis affects you. The following general guidelines can help you assess this, as will talking to your doctor and/or physiotherapist.

To see how fit you are, think about the following:

- if you do a minimum of three sessions of aerobic exercise a week, you are *fit*
- if you do a minimum of one aerobic session a week or have an active lifestyle (for example, you do lots of gardening, brisk continuous walking, going up and down stairs), you are *moderately fit*
- if you are any less active than the above, you are *unfit*.

Thinking about the following points will help you assess how arthritis affects your daily life. Does it mean:

- no noticeable affect on your ability to do your usual tasks
- you can do the tasks, but there is some discomfort and mobility is affected

- you find tasks such as dressing and bathing very difficult and need help
- your movement is very restricted, you are bedridden or wheelchair-bound.

Armed with your assessment of your fitness and arthritis, remind yourself of what an exercise programme for people with arthritis should do. It should:

- reduce and relieve any discomfort, stiffness, and pain
- prevent further disability, deformity, deterioration
- give you more energy to perform your daily tasks
- increase your self-esteem, confidence and enjoyment of life.

Getting started

Prepare your exercise area:

- make the room in which you exercise as pleasant as possible
- have equipment (chair, weights, bands and so on) handy
- have drinking water nearby
- have two towels – one rolled to use as a cushion under your head, hips or buttocks, the other to mop your brow
- take the phone off the hook
- wear loose, comfortable clothes.

Several things may slow down beginners: remembering what to do, when and how to do it, and keeping track of the number of repetitions.

To start with, you will find yourself glancing at the instructions frequently, trying to get the positions right, and finding it hard to remember which exercise comes next. If you exercise regularly, though, it is amazing how quickly you can begin to memorize the routines. In the meantime, try to put the book in a convenient place, where you can see it easily.

You do not have to hold positions for precisely the length of time given, but the recommended effective limit for all exercises in this book is six seconds. You will soon begin to sense how long this is without looking at your watch or clock.

Counting repetitions can be a nuisance. Most people can manage to count up to five repetitions with little difficulty; after that, ingenuity may be needed. Try speaking out loud, learn to listen to your body, and take a pride in your technique.

Before you start the exercises a final, encouraging, thought. Remember that when you bought this book, you took a decision to do something more to help your arthritis. Now, each time you exercise, you are taking an important step towards being more in control.

How the exercise programme works

We have divided the exercises into activity segments or blocks. These can be put together in any combination that suits you. How you do this will depend on how much time you have, what you want to work on that day, your state of health, and so on. For example, if you have an hour and are in a good state of health, you could do *all* the blocks. However, if you are short of time or in discomfort, you may simply do the warm-up and cool-down blocks. Use the following chart to help guide you.

The exercise programme

Activity block	Duration
Block 1 – Warm-up Muscle warming	5 minutes
Block 2 – Warm-up Mobility and stretching	10 minutes
Block 3 Strengthening	15 minutes

Block 4 Aerobic	Low level: 5 minutes Moderate level: 10–15 minutes Moderate to low level: 5 minutes
Block 5 – Cool-down Mobility and stretches from Block 2	5 minutes

Note: You must *always* do the warm-up and cool-down blocks.

When planning your week, the following chart can help you decide when and how often to exercise. It is only a guide, so be considerate and listen to your body. There will be times when you will be unable to reach your planned target, but do not worry, simply do whichever mobility exercises feel comfortable. If this is too much, then concentrate on posture and relaxation instead.

Type of Exercise	Sessions per Week	Intensity
Mobility	5–7	Low to moderate
Flexibility	5	Low to moderate
Muscle strength	2–3	Low to moderate
Aerobic	2–4	Low to moderate
Balance, co-ordination	5	Low to moderate
Posture	7	Not applicable

Keeping going

Starting to exercise may not be too difficult. You will be full of enthusiasm. Aware of the likely benefits, you probably cannot wait to get started. Although you will feel better almost immediately, it will take time before you notice the physical differences – the increased range of movement and strength, a lessening of pain, more energy. In the meantime, you will only experience these benefits if you motivate yourself to keep exercising regularly. Then, when you do begin to feel better and stronger, you may be tempted to think that you do not have to continue to exercise. Be warned – as soon as you give up, the benefits begin to slip away. So, be determined!

Often people reach a sort of plateau, a time when you may feel you have made some progress, but everything seems to have come to a halt. If this happens, you may need to make slight adjustments to your routine, say, trying a different series of exercises, finding a new environment or taking up a new activity.

Remember, the benefits of exercise are measurable:

- shoulder movements become larger and easier
- arms can be lifted higher with more control
- legs become stronger and more stable
- breathing during activity is deeper, more even
- you can do more, and for longer, with more energy
- you will stand taller and straighter as your posture improves
- your balance and co-ordination will be better
- you will react faster and more skilfully
- you may be more resistant to infections
- you will cope with stress better
- quality of sleep improves
- you will feel more positive and relaxed.

How to motivate yourself

Think about:

- the risks of *not* experiencing the benefits of exercise
- the financial and emotional costs of being dependent on others
- the disappointment you will feel if you do not take this opportunity or if you drop out.

Decide how often you will exercise and for how long. The routines are very adaptable. You can pick just a handful of movements to do every day, two or three times a day, particularly for mobility or you can choose to do a longer routine, once a day or three or four times a week.

Some people find it helpful to make a timetable and slot in their exercise session. It often helps to have a definite time that you know you will devote to your exercise. Think of it rather like a business or doctor's appointment, as something that cannot be altered. In order to do this successfully, you could make out a check-list for each day over the course of a week, writing in the exercises in the most appropriate spaces.

Other people prefer to be a little bit more flexible and allot a certain time of day or evening to exercising, being prepared to give or take an hour or so either way. If you put yourself under pressure regarding your exercises, you will benefit less as you may spend too much time worrying about getting things absolutely right.

Most people do seem to need some sort of routine, no matter how simple. This is because, psychologically, if you think of your exercise routine as an integral part of the day – as important as getting dressed, brushing your teeth, eating a meal – you will find it easier to make it part of your life. This is why it makes sense to do something that is connected with exercise each day of the week, and this includes your relaxation routine.

Do not be too tough on yourself, though. If there is a change of plan that means there is no time for exercise on one of your days, take this in your stride. However, be honest with yourself and see whether perhaps it is possible to move the things you want to do around and still make time for exercise.

If you feel you are losing interest remember:
- never say quit – for more than a day!
- do not let a slip turn into a slide
- reward yourself for keeping at it – after 1, 3, 6, and 12 months
- it's never too late to begin again.

The exercises

What follows is a pot-pourri of safe and effective chair and standing exercises. You can either follow the order given or mix and match, according to how your body (and, in particular, your joints) are feeling. Try also to alternate between exercises for the upper and lower body, such as shoulders and knees.

Remember

Always do a warm-up and cool-down session (Blocks 1 and 2) and avoid mixing exercises from different blocks.

The exercise basics

Your exercise chair

It has no arms.
It has a straight back, and the back is high enough to hold from behind without stooping.
It has a firm seat.
The seat height is at just the right height so that when you sit on it, your feet are flat on the ground.

The pelvic tilt

Place your body weight in correct alignment.
For safe and effective standing, lying and sitting.
Do it all day, every day, everywhere.

Tilt your pelvis, bringing your lower back under, your hip-bones and pelvis forward.
Pull in your tummy muscles to secure the position.
Breathe in as you tighten the tummy, and out as you relax.

Posture: sit or stand tall

Feel the difference in your body, mind, and attitude.

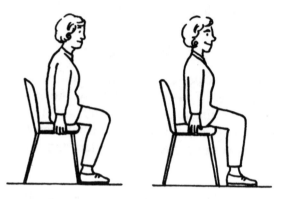

SITTING Sit on your chair, then lift yourself slightly away from the back of your chair so that you are *sitting tall*. Make sure your legs and feet are hip width apart, and your knees are over your ankles, not tucked under the chair.

Do a pelvic tilt.
Lift your ribs up away from your waist.
Press your shoulders down and back.
Lengthen the back of your neck upwards and keep your jaw parallel to the floor.
Let your arms hang loosely at your sides.

STANDING Stand with your feet hip width apart, toes slightly outwards and knees over your toes. Soften your knees.

Do a pelvic tilt and tighten the tummy muscles.
Lift the ribs up away from the waist.
Press your shoulders down and back.
Keeping your jaw horizontal, lengthen the back of the neck upwards and keep your jaw parallel to the floor.
Let your arms hang loosely at your sides.

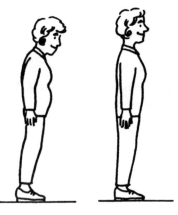

CHECKPOINTS Check that your:

- bottom is under
- chest is lifted
- your tummy muscles are tightened
- your spine has lengthened.

Warm-up

Checkpoints to remember when you do your warm-up.

- Check that your posture is correct before, and several times during, the exercises.
- Focus on the pelvic tilt and tightening your tummy muscles.
- Make all arm and leg movements in a controlled and rhythmical way.
- When you are exercising sitting on your chair, never lift both legs at once. Hold your chair seat to support your back, unless you are working your legs and arms in opposite directions.
- Breathe easily throughout.
- Feel your muscles getting warmer and more pliable as you increase your circulation.

Block 1 – Warm-up: muscle-warming

Clap, swing warmer

Combine some clapping and low arm swings. Prepare by improving your posture, sitting or standing tall.

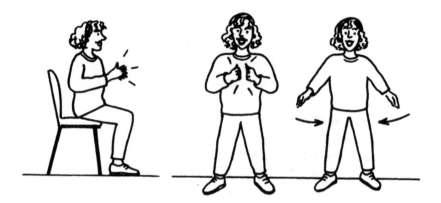

Make six claps on your thighs.
Make six claps at waist height.
Rest your hands on your thighs or hips.
Repeat four times.
Sway your arms across your body, from right to left, four times. Rest.
Repeat all this six times, getting into a rhythm that feels good to you.

CHECKPOINTS Check that your:

- posture is correct throughout, and breathe easily
- body is getting warmer.

Swing warmer

Prepare by improving your posture, sitting or standing tall.

EXERCISE, REST AND RELAXATION

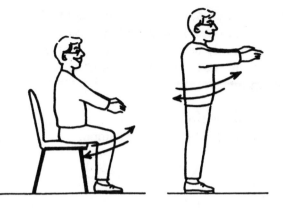

Take both your arms forwards, from the seat of your chair to just above the knees, in one low swing.

Turn your wrists and lower arms to sides of thighs.

Repeat four times.

Rest then repeat the movements six times, getting into a rhythm.

CHECKPOINTS Check that you are:

- breathing easily
- getting warmer.

Easy walking

Prepare by sitting or standing tall with your feet close together.

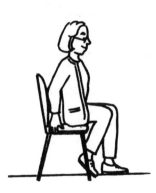 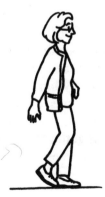

Lift one heel and then the other, taking the weight slowly from one foot to the other in a 'pedalling' action, keeping the weight distributed evenly between both feet. Roll the weight through each foot from the toe to the heel and back.
Repeat ten times.
Rest.
Repeat the above twice.
For *chairwork*: hold the seat for support.

CHECKPOINTS Check that your:

● posture is correct throughout.

Room walking
Progress from Easy walking to 'travelling' by walking around the room.

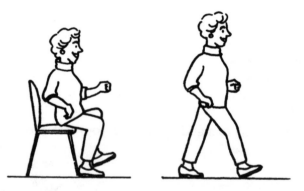

Start with small, short strides and gradually build up to a moderate pace. Transfer the weight evenly and build up to an enjoyable rhythm.
Keep your arms low and move them in the opposite direction to your legs.
Do about ten of these, then Easy walk again.
Repeat six times.

For *chairwork*: simulate walking by lifting first one knee and then the other.

Marching and baby rocking

Keeping your movements slow and low, stand tall and march on the spot ten times.

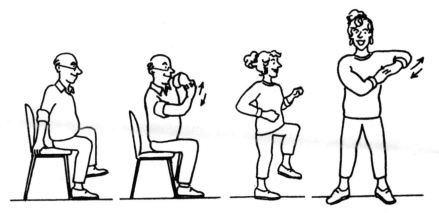

Swing your arms in the opposite direction to your legs.
For *chairwork* hold the seat while moving your legs.
Then, standing, with your feet shoulder width apart, your hips facing forwards, sway from side to side ten times.
(For chair and standing:)
Link your fingers together or lay one arm across the other and sway your arms across your body as though you were rocking a baby to sleep.
Repeat the sequence four times.

Torvill and Dean

Pretend you are ice skating on the spot, coming forwards and transferring your weight from leg to leg.
Sway your arms as if rocking a baby to sleep as before eight times.
Repeat the skating action, backwards this time, keeping your hips facing forwards, eight times.
Repeat the sequence four times.

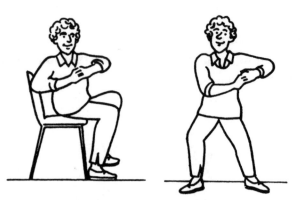

Block 2 – Warm-up: mobility and stretching
You need to do these exercises to:

- regain and maintain your joints' full natural ranges of movement
- realign your joints correctly
- improve your posture, which will help you do everyday tasks more easily.

Checkpoints to remember when you do your mobilizing and stretching exercises
- Always do the muscle-warmer first.
- Do mobilizing exercises daily if at all possible, plus the chest, shoulder and back stretches and body lengthener exercises on pages 59-62, five to seven times a week.
- Try three to five repetitions of each exercise, unless your joints are vulnerable. If so, try one or two repetitions.
- Make your movements in a slow and controlled way.
- Always work to your full, natural range of movement, but never to the point where it is painful.
- If you experience pain, *stop*. If pain persists or recurs, *stop*. If you have sudden, sharp pain, seek medical advice.
- Check with your doctor *before* doing these exercises, particularly if you have had joint surgery or if your arthritis is severe.

- When you do the exercises regularly notice the differences they make in your daily life, to your ability to bend to pick things up, dress yourself, comb your hair and so on.

Shoulder mobilizer

These two movements feel good and will loosen and lubricate the joints, helping you to maintain a good range of movement, to release tension in your neck and shoulders, and prevent a rounded back.

Prepare by improving your posture, sitting or standing tall.

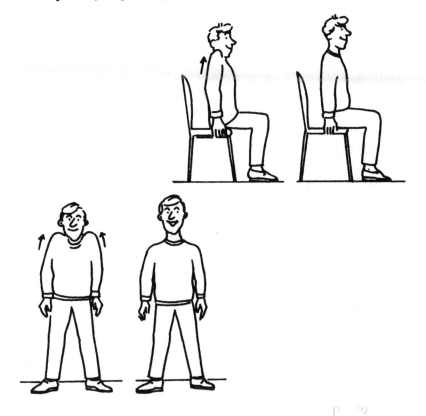

Lift your shoulders up lightly, then draw them down, away from the ears.

Repeat four times.

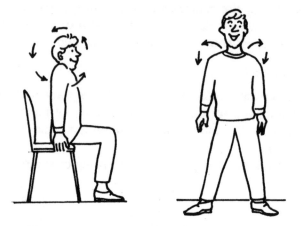

Roll your shoulders forwards, upwards, backwards and down.
Hold them in the back and down position for a moment, then
move the shoulders in a continuous circle, moving smoothly and
slowly.
Rest.
Repeat four times.

Ankle mobilizer

You will really feel and see a difference if you do these regularly.
Your ankle stiffness will reduce and your ankles will feel looser,
especially when you step and stride and go up and down stairs.
Breathe easily throughout.

Prepare by improving your posture, sitting or standing tall.

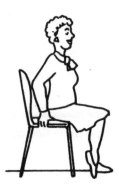

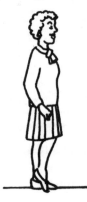

Stand near a wall or the back of your exercise chair and use them to support you.

Bend one knee slightly, to support your weight safely.

With the other foot, put first the heel, then the toe on the floor in a heel-to-toe action.

Repeat the up and down movement slowly and deliberately, gradually increasing the range of movement of your ankle joint.

ALTERNATIVELY Sit on your exercise chair, quite far forward, and support your body by holding the chair seat with both hands. Take your weight on one leg as you put first the heel and then the toe of your other foot on the floor.

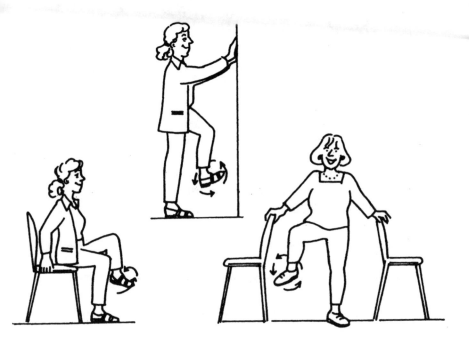

Prepare and support your weight as above.

Slowly circle your foot first clockwise, then anticlockwise.

Rest and repeat with your other ankle.

Repeat three times each side.

Upper back mobilizer

This exercise mobilizes the middle and upper parts of the spine and is very important for good posture and efficient lung function. Feel your spine become looser, your chest more open and your back stronger – and feel the lift in your spirits!

Prepare by improving your posture, sitting and standing tall.

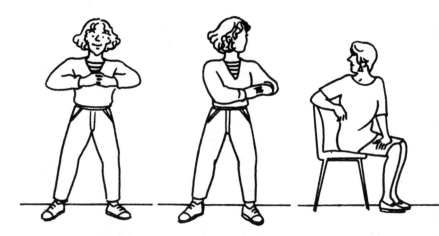

Stand, legs hip width apart, with your elbows bent at chest level and forearms resting against each other.

Do a pelvic tilt, tightening your tummy and keeping hips facing forward.

Turn your upper body to the side and take your head round to look behind you.

Repeat, turning to the other side, four times on each side.

ALTERNATIVELY Sit on your exercise chair and turn your upper body as above.

Take the arm across the back of the chair.

Place the other arm across your knees and, keeping your hips facing forwards, gently ease your upper body round to look behind you. Move your head round as well so that you are looking over your shoulder.

Hold the position for a moment.
Repeat, turning to the other side.

Knee and hip mobilizer

Prepare by improving your posture, sitting or standing tall.

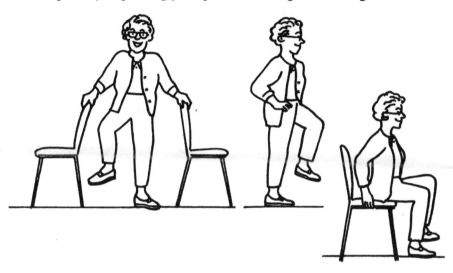

HIP Start by slowly lifting your heel straight up off the floor so that your knee lifts up, bends, and your hip flexes.
Alternate your left and right legs, repeating this ten times each side.
Build up the size of the movement you make until you can balance well and can lift your knee as high as is comfortable. Make sure your chest is lifted and your posture is good.

KNEE This second exercise loosens the knee joint and is a great one to do every 15 minutes or so if you have to sit or stand for long periods. Breathe easily throughout.
    Prepare by improving your posture, sitting or standing tall.

Use a wall or the back of your exercise chair to support you until you can stand balancing with your hands on your hips.
Start by slowly lifting your heel towards your bottom. Make

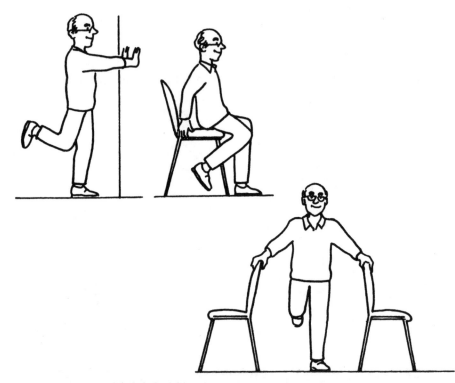

sure your thigh is held backwards away from the hip and that you keep it still – do not allow it to swing forwards. Avoid arching your back as you do this.

Repeat, alternating left and right legs.

Build up the size of movement gradually.

Perform the exercise slowly and carefully, and concentrate on controlling the leg when you return the foot to the floor.

ALTERNATIVELY Sit on your exercise chair holding the seat with both hands, and bend the knee backwards under the chair as above.

Middle and upper back mobilizer

This will improve your range of movement.

Prepare by improving your posture, sitting or standing tall.

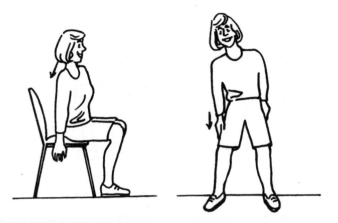

Either on your exercise chair or standing, slide one hand down your thigh, keeping your neck and back in a straight line. Do not lean backwards or forwards as you do this.

Hold the position for two to three seconds, then return to the starting position.

Repeat on the other side.

Lower back mobilizer and lengthener

These exercises are a wonderful way to care for your back. They loosen the lower spine, release tension and can ease back pain.

Put one hand on your lower back and the other on your tummy while you do the exercises and you will feel your spine moving.

Prepare by improving your posture, sitting or standing tall.

Do a pelvic tilt, then bring your bottom even further forwards, bringing your hip bones up towards your nose.

Slowly move back to the starting position until you are sitting or standing tall again.

Repeat eight times, then rest.

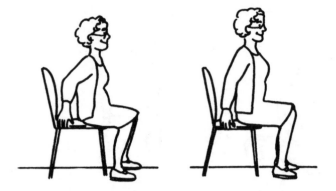

Hip and spine mobilizer

Standing, or sitting on your exercise chair, standing or sitting tall, tighten your tummy muscles and lift one hip up towards your ribs.

Lower it, then repeat on the other side.

Repeat several times.

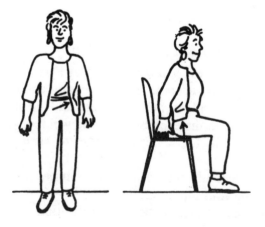

Wrist mobilizer

Prepare by improving your posture, sitting or standing tall.

Bend your arms at the elbows.

Tuck your elbows into your waist and hold your lower arms out in front, at right angles to your elbows, with your palms facing each other.

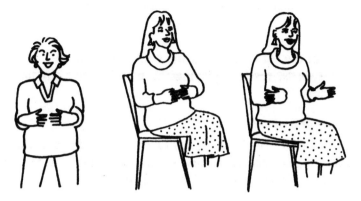

Bring your fingertips towards each other, bending only at the wrists. Keep your hands straight and take your fingertips as far inwards as possible.

Reverse the movement, keeping your arms and wrists still and taking the fingers as far apart as possible.

Repeat four times.

Rest.

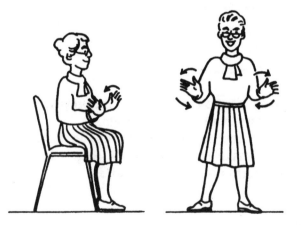

Adopt the same position as above.

Bring your fingertips towards each other as before, but this time, move your hands in circles from the wrists – up, in, out, down.

Repeat four times.

Rest.

Repeat, making circles in the opposite direction.
Rest.

Repeat the series of flexes and circles once more.
Afterwards, rest by 'playing the piano' with your fingers and thumbs.

Finger mobilizer

If you find you have difficulty with your fingers during this exercise, exercise each hand separately, using your free hand to gently assist the fingers of the other hand.

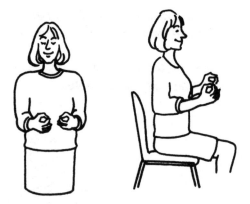

Adopt the same position as you did for the previous exercise, but hold your elbows loosely at waist height.
Touch the tip of each finger to the thumb (on the same hand) in turn trying to make round, large 'O' shapes in space. Then stretch the fingers out into a wide V after.
Then rest.

Neck mobilizers

The following two exercises are best done when the body has warmed up a little and any neck tension has been released by previous exercises. Always do these exercises slowly and in a controlled way.
   Prepare by improving your posture, sitting or standing tall.

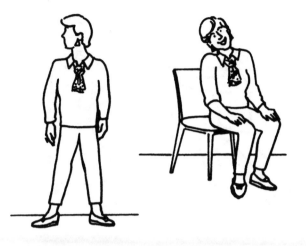

Look straight ahead and lengthen the back of your neck.
Turn your head and look over your shoulder.
Hold for two to three seconds and return to starting position.
Lengthen your neck once more and repeat to other side.
Build up the degree of movement in your neck until you are
looking as far over your shoulder as possible.

Keep looking straight ahead, lengthening your neck and keeping
your jaw parallel with the floor throughout.
Tilt your head down towards your shoulder, feel the neck
loosening and lengthening on the opposite side of your neck.
Hold the position for two to three seconds.
Lift your head back up to the centre again.
Repeat on the other side and do this four times each side.

Hip stretch

This is a daily must as it counteracts the negative effects of sitting,
helping to give back length to shortened muscles and increasing
the range of movement in the hips.

Stand tall, facing the back of your exercise chair or wall – use this
for support during the exercise.

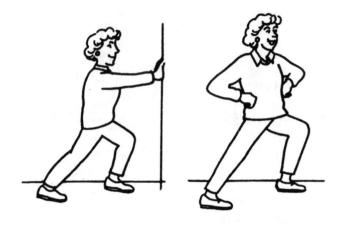

With your legs hip width apart, move one leg a step back, feet facing forwards, bend your front leg. Keep the back leg straight with your heel on the floor. Then bring your bottom under and your hips forwards and upwards. As you tilt your pelvis, you will feel a strong stretching sensation in the front of the hip of your back leg. Hold for a count of ten.

Ease slowly into and out of this stretch.

Have an 'active' rest, circling your hips gently.

Repeat on the opposite side.

Calf stretch

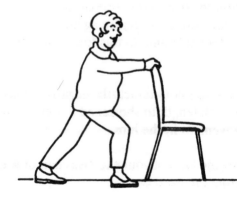

This will put a spring in your step and length in your stride!

Adopt the same position as for the previous exercise.

Do a pelvic tilt for good posture and take the weight forward very slightly. Keep your heels on the floor, and feel the stretch in the calf muscle of the leg behind.

Check the posture of your upper body, think tall, and hold for a count of ten.

Bring your back leg to the front again, walk on the spot to loosen your legs, then repeat on the other side.

Repeat four times each side.

Hamstring stretch

Another essential daily exercise, this maintains a full range of movement at the hip and makes putting on trousers, doing up shoelaces and a host of other daily tasks much easier.

Prepare by improving your posture, sitting tall near the edge of your exercise chair.

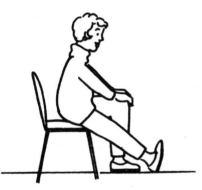

Straighten one leg out in front of you, resting your heel on the floor.

Place both hands on the opposite knee to support your back and bodyweight.

Sit tall.

Lean your upper body forward an upward until you feel a stretch in the muscles at the back of your thigh (your hamstring). Hold for a count of ten.

Have an 'active' rest, wriggling your shoulders and hips to release any tension.
Repeat on the other side.
Repeat four times each side.

Inner thigh stretch
If you have had hip or knee surgery, do not do this exercise.

This makes everyday walking, climbing onto buses, etc., much easier. It will help to lengthen your stride.
   Prepare by improving your posture, sitting tall either on the floor or your exercise chair.

Support yourself either with your hands at sides of the seat of the chair or behind you on the floor.

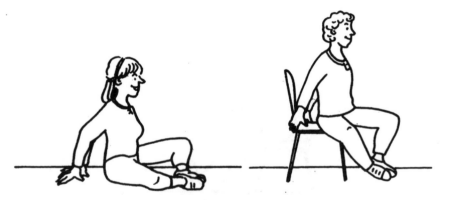

Place the soles of your feet together and allow your knees to fall away from each other towards the floor.
Pressing on your hands, gently ease your knees further towards the floor until you feel a stretch along your inner thighs. Hold for a count of ten.
Place your hands on your knees and ease gently down for an extra stretch, but do *not* do this if your arthritis is severe.

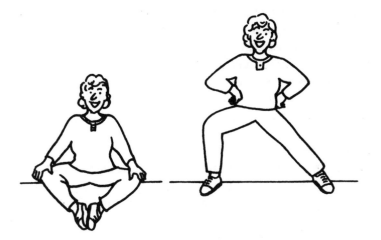

You can also stretch your inner thighs standing, with or without support.

Take one leg out to the side, your hips facing forwards. Bend one leg slightly over your toes and keep your other leg straight, but not locked at the knee and foot flat on the floor. You will feel a stretch along your inner thigh. If you can't feel the stretch, go back to the start and take a wider step to the side.

Chest stretch

This is great for curing rounded shoulders, improving your breathing, and it gives you an immediate release of energy.

Prepare by improving your posture, sitting tall.

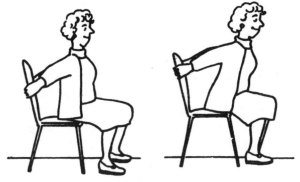

On your exercise chair, sit with your legs hip width apart.
Hold on to the back of the chair with both hands.
Let your arms lengthen as you lean slowly forwards. Keep your
ribs lifted, head up, jaw horizontal, shoulders down. Hold for a
count of ten.
Feel the stretch across the chest and arms and the strengthening
in your upper back.

Shoulder and back stretch

This will help you to continue to do up zips, buttons, scratch your
back, pull jumpers on and off with ease.
   Prepare by improving your posture, sitting or standing tall.

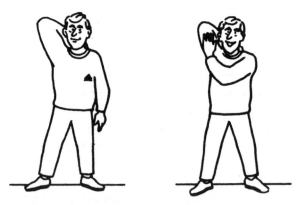

Lift your right arm straight up towards the ceiling. Then, bending
your arm at the elbow, bring your hand as far down your back as
possible.
Take your other arm across your chest and support the raised
arm. Now, ease your bent arm up and back until you feel a
stretch along the front of the upper arm. If you feel discomfort or
your arthritis is severe, take this very easy. Alternatively bring
the arm across the chest and ease it in towards the chest with the
other arm. If you are very flexible, take your other arm up over
your head and hold your bent arm just above the elbow.

Body lengthener

This will keep your body tall and improve your posture.
Prepare by sitting or standing tall.

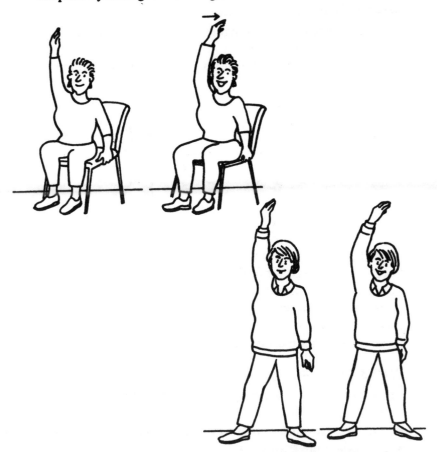

Lift one arm up towards the ceiling, and extending up out of the
ribs as far as possible, keeping the shoulder down.

Breathe out and take your extended arm slightly over your head,
feeling a stretch down your side. Keep your ribs lifted, your back
long, your tummy muscles tight and your other shoulder down
and relaxed.

Change arms and repeat as many times as is comfortable. If your arthritis is severe, simply rest the palm of your hand on your shoulder and lift your elbow as high as you can or do this with your hands at your sides.

Wrist and finger stretch

This helps prevent your fingers curling in. Do the exercise as often as feels comfortable.

Prepare by improving your posture, sitting or standing tall.

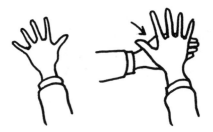

Spread your fingers out wide and flat, as though spanning piano keys. Hold for a count of six.

Spread your fingers out wide as before and place the palm of your other hand across them, avoiding the fingertips. Press lightly and hold for a count of ten.

Repeat twice, then do the same with your other hand.

Block 3: Strengthening exercises

These exercises are important because they help:

- improve the muscles that support the joints
- strengthen the bones
- improve posture and the functioning of the body
- help you do everyday tasks more easily.

Checkpoints to remember when you are doing your strengthening exercises

- Try to do two or three non-consecutive days of strengthening exercises a week.

- On difficult days, do just one repetition.
- When holding a position, do not hold your breath as well – keep breathing easily throughout.
- When holding a position, never hold it for longer than a count of six as your blood pressure may begin to rise a little.
- Start slowly and progress gradually. Do the exercises for about a month before progressing to the next stage.

Equipment

The equipment you need to do the following exercises does not have to be expensive.

- You can buy stretchy bands, but support tights tied together at the ends are a cheap substitute (or you can use old bicycle inner tubes when you are stronger).
- Dyna-band and Thera-band are ideal if you want to buy stretchy bands as they are specially designed and come in different strengths and colours for you to change to as you progress.
- Always tie bands with a bow rather than a knot as they are easier to undo.
- Home-made weights can be bags of rice, sand, sugar, flour or similar. If you want to buy some, they come in various colours and different weights – begin with 0.5 kg (1 lb 2 oz) and increase the weight you use as you become fitter, but do not exceed 2 kg (4½ lb)
- Have your equipment ready before you begin to exercise.

Side of shoulder strengthener

Prepare by improving your posture, sitting or standing tall, and putting a weight in your hand.

Keeping your elbow slightly bent, raise your arm out to the side to shoulder level.
Slowly lower your arm to the starting position.
Repeat until your arm begins to tire.
Rest and repeat on the other side.

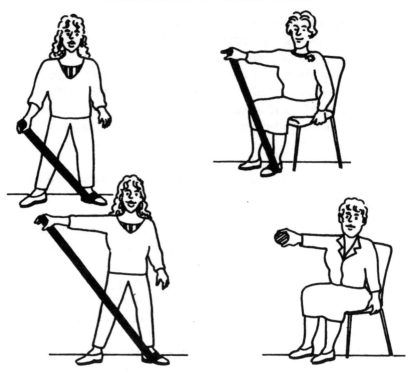

Rest actively by shrugging your shoulders.

Repeat once more on each side, feeling the muscle working at the top and side of your shoulder.

Keep a good pelvic tilt and tighten tummy muscles throughout.

Shoulder and arm rowing

This exercise will really help straighten rounded shoulders and lessen strain on the upper spine. It also opens the chest and increases the range of movement of the shoulders.

Prepare by improving your posture, sitting or standing tall, and putting a weight in your hand.

Keeping your elbow slightly bent, take your whole arm up and back as if you were rowing.

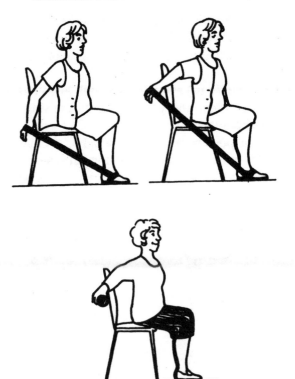

Hold your arm at the furthest point for one second, then slowly lower your arm to the starting position at the side of the ribs. Rest for two seconds, then repeat the exercise until you feel tired.

Rest.

Repeat on the other side, feeling the muscles working at the top and back of your shoulder and in your upper back.

After this, rest actively by shrugging your shoulders to loosen any tightness.

Back of arm strengthener

When toned, this much-neglected muscle will help you to lift heavier objects more safely, especially those from high cupboards and so on. The exercise will help the muscle to

support the shoulder joint and strengthen the bones in the shoulder and arm and it takes away that wobbly look from the underarm!
Prepare by improving your posture, sitting or standing tall.

Stand about 15 cm (6 in) away from a wall, arms out in front of you at shoulder height and your palms on the wall, directly in front of your shoulders.
Check that your posture is good, do a pelvic tilt and keep your tummy muscles pulled in to avoid arching your back, then slowly bend your elbows to lower your body towards the wall.

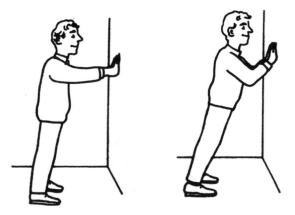

Push yourself slowly back to the starting position.
Repeat six times, breathing easily throughout.
Rest actively, shrugging your shoulders and shaking your wrists.
Repeat.
As this becomes easier, increase your fitness by placing your palms further apart. After several months, take another step away from the wall.

ALTERNATIVELY Sit tall on your exercise chair and hold tins of baked beans or other weights in your hands.

Check your posture.
Take your arms and shoulders down and back as far as possible.
Bend your arms so that your lower arms are at right angles to

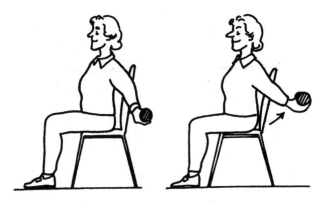

your upper arms and hold your upper arms against your ribs.
Your palms should be facing upwards.
Straighten out your lower arms, so that your palms and the
weights in them are facing the ceiling. Hold for a second. Then
lower the arm to a right angle.
Repeat six times.
Rest actively, rolling and shrugging your shoulders and wrists.
Repeat three times.

Wrist wring

This is wonderful for weak wrists. It strengthens them and
will make unscrewing jars and pots much easier!
   Prepare by improving your posture, sitting or standing tall,
and holding a towel or rubber mat between your hands.

Make squeezing and wringing movements, as if you were trying
to get rid of as much water as possible. Do this first in one
direction, then the other until your wrists begin to tire.
Rest actively shaking your wrists and rolling your neck gently
from side to side. (*Never* roll neck to the back.)
Repeat four times.

ALTERNATIVELY Rest your arms on your thighs. Using a small

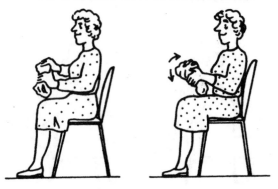

towel rolled into a ball or tennis balls, squeeze and release until you tire.
Repeat four times.

Chest press

Prepare by improving your posture, sitting or standing tall. Use either weights or a stretchy band for this exercise, putting the weights in your hands or the band round your upper back with the ends in your hands, pulling it taut.

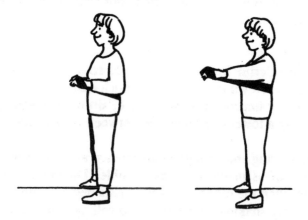

With your palms facing downwards, bend your elbows, tucking them in against your waist, and hold your lower arms at right angles to your body.
Straighten your arms out in front to just below shoulder height

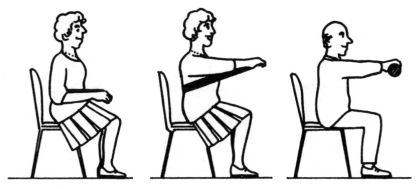

(your arms will then be parallel with the floor). Hold for a second.

Slowly bend your elbows until you return to the right angle and, finally, lower them slightly.

Take care to keep your tummy muscles tight, your back long, and your knees soft (slightly bent) as you do the exercise.

Feel the muscles working in your chest.

Shrug and wriggle your shoulders to release any tension.

Repeat twice.

Back and rear shoulder strengthener

This is one of the most effective exercises there is for straightening out rounded shoulders. It also helps to reduce the pressure on the joints, and greatly increases the range of movement and strength of the muscles in both your shoulders and back.

If this feels uncomfortable or too strong for you, then continue to do the exercise without weights or a band.

Prepare by sitting or standing tall and holding weights in your hands or a stretchy band in front of your chest.

Check that your posture is good.

Draw your shoulders and elbows back towards your spine, pulling your shoulder blades together, and hold for a count of three. Feel the muscles working at the backs of your shoulders and in your upper back.

Take your arms back to the starting position.

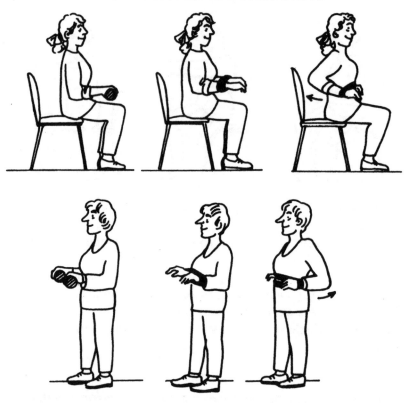

Repeat six times.

Rest actively by shrugging and wriggling your shoulders to release any tension.

Leg press

This exercise stabilizes the knee joint by working the thigh muscle that helps the knee to track correctly. Indeed, many knee problems can be caused because of poor tone in this muscle. Do this and the next exercise for the maximum beneficial effect.

Prepare by improving your posture, sitting tall on your exercise chair with your legs together. Loop a stretchy band once around the instep of your foot, keep it taut and hold the ends securely under your hands, resting the palms on the sides of the seat of the chair.

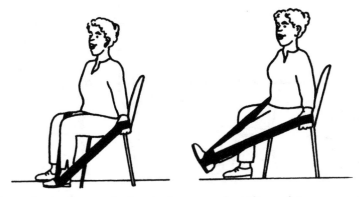

Extend your leg out in front of you, against the resistance exerted by the band. Move smoothly and take care to avoid locking the knee. Hold the position for two seconds. Feel the muscle in the front of your thigh working.

Return to your starting position and repeat until your muscles begin to tire.

Standing leg strengthener

This helps you to maintain your independence and mobility.

Prepare by improving your posture, sitting tall at the front of your exercise chair.

Really tighten your tummy muscles.

Prepare to move after a slow count of three.

Keeping your head up throughout, lean forwards to take the weight over your hips and let your thighs do all the work as you stand up.

Stand tall.

Steady yourself, then reverse the movement by keeping your body upright, bending your knees, then lowering yourself slowly and carefully back onto the chair. Feel the muscles in the front and back of your thighs and buttocks working.

To start with, you may wish to place your hands on your thighs (*not* on the chair) to help you get up and sit down, but gradually lessen the pressure until you are just relying on leg power.

71

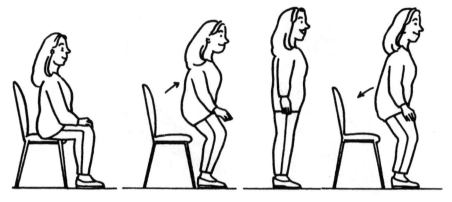

Calf raises

Prepare by improving your posture, standing tall.

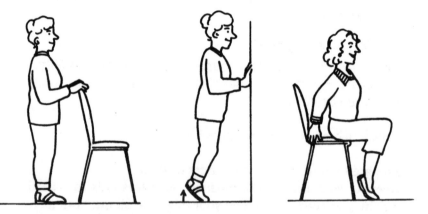

Stand, facing the back of your exercise chair or a wall. Check that your posture is good.

Take your bodyweight slightly forwards, lifting your heels up and rising on the ball of your foot as far as you can.

Lower yourself back to your starting position with control. Make sure you shift the weight gradually right through the foot, from heel to toe and back again. Keep the weight mainly on your big toe and second toe, and avoid putting weight on your little toe.

Repeat until your calves begin to tire.
Walk on the spot to release the tension that builds up in the calf muscles.

If this feels too strong, do extra Ankle mobilizer (see page 46) and leg strengthener (see page 71) exercises until your legs and feet are stronger.

Standing hip strengthener

This exercise helps you increase the range of movement of your hips and strengthens your buttock muscles so you can take unnecessary weight and strain off the hip joint.

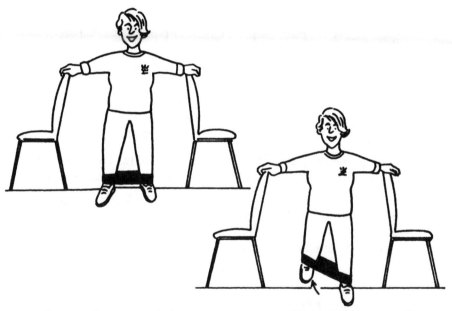

Prepare by improving your posture, standing tall. Face a wall or stand between two sturdy chairs, then either loop and secure a stretchy band around your ankles or tie small bags of rice or sand round them.

If you are using a wall to support you, stand with your feet about 10 cm (4 ins) away from it with your arms out in front of you at shoulder height and your palms resting on the wall.

If you are using chairs to support you, hold on to them to balance yourself.

Make sure your weight is evenly distributed between both legs, check that your posture is good, your tummy muscles are tight, and keep your knees slightly bent throughout, then prepare to move after a slow count of three.

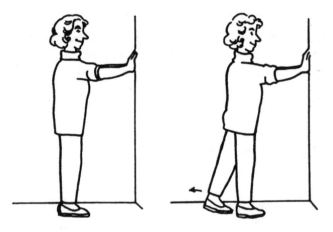

Keeping one foot in place try to press the other leg backwards along the floor as far as possible. (You may lift the leg a little as you do this but think of going *back* rather than *up*.) The movement will be small, but controlled.

Hold your position at the furthest point for a count of six.

Return to your starting position, then repeat with your other leg.

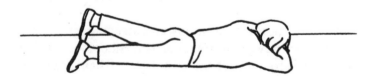

ALTERNATIVELY Lie face down on the floor, with or without the band or weights, and make the same movement. Never lift *both* legs.

Hip opener and strengthener

Prepare by improving your posture, sitting or standing tall, with your feet and legs 5 cm (2 ins) apart.

You will need the same equipment as for the previous exercise.

Prepare to move by counting to three, and tighten your tummy muscles.

Using your arms to support you and keeping one foot in place, try to press the other leg sideways along the floor – just as far as you can without your hip lifting. Keep your knee and toes facing forwards, your ankle leading the sideways movement. Your leg and foot will lift a little, but think of going along the floor *sideways* rather than *up*.

Make the movement in a slow, controlled way, feeling the muscle in the outside of the hip and buttock working.

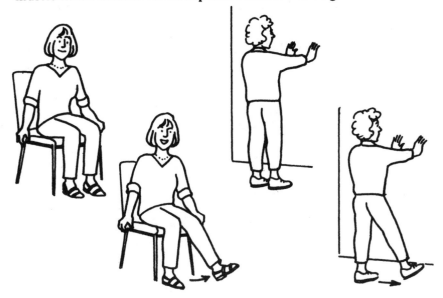

ALTERNATIVELY Sitting with your back supported against a wall and pillow for comfort. Prepare as before and take the legs

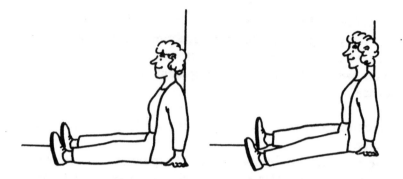

slowly apart about ten inches. Keep legs in contact with the floor throughout and the tummy tight to support the back.

Tummy and upper body strengthener

These two exercises, as well as making your tummy flatter, are vital in order to improve posture and help protect your back. You can do them any time, anywhere, and soon feel and see the difference!

Follow the breathing instructions and do not come up too far, too fast.

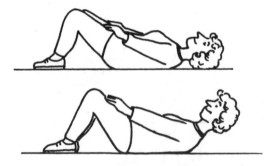

Lie on your back with your legs hip width apart. Bend your knees and place feet flat on floor. Rest your palms on the fronts of your thighs. Check your posture, ensuring that your back is long and pressed into the floor and your tummy muscles are tightened.

76

Lift your shoulders off the floor as you slide your fingers up towards your knees, making sure your neck is long so that there is a good space between your chin and chest. Breathe out as you come up and pull your tummy in, and breathe in as you lower. Lower yourself slowly and with control back down to the floor. Repeat five times.
Rest.
Repeat three times.
If you neck is uncomfortable support it with one hand.

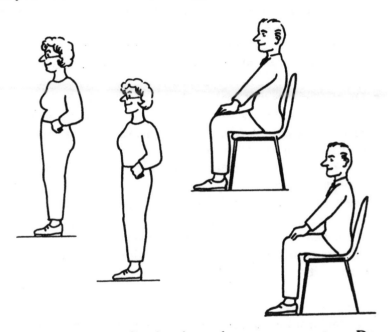

Either *sitting or standing* bend your knees over your toes. Do a pelvic tilt, check your posture, and tighten your tummy muscles. Pull your tummy in really hard towards your spine while allowing it to curve under a little. Keep your chest lifted and relaxed. Hold for a count of six.
Release.
Repeat ten times.
Rest.
Repeat three times.

Block 4

These exercises are vital for a healthy heart and lungs. They are like the exercises from Block 1, but the movements are bigger, more vigorous and more energetic. They are aerobic i.e. need oxygen to perform them.

Checkpoints to remember when you are doing your aerobic exercises

- Always do a warm-up session first and a cool-down session after these exercises.
- Build up and ease down gradually, making a quarter of your session low; half of your session moderate to hard; and a quarter moderate to low intensity.
- Do movements that use your legs and arms rhythmically.
- Never stop suddenly, always ease down, making your movements gradually smaller, until you are walking, gradually slowing down to a stop.
- Wherever possible, exercise on carpet, grass or some other springy surface.
- Wear loose, comfortable clothes, suitable footwear, preferably with shock-absorbing soles. Never work in just socks.
- Have water nearby to drink during and after.
- Discuss your intended programme with your doctor *before* starting it.

Clap swings

Make big arm movements, clapping at waist, chest, and head level, and overhead.

Make your whole body sway as you swing your arms across your body, from right to left, to waist, shoulder, and, finally, head height. Perform all sways and swings with control.

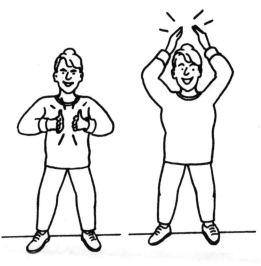

Swing turns

Sitting on your exercise chair, swing your arms forwards, building up to bigger and bigger movements, from hip-high swings to shoulder to head-high, even swinging yourself up off the chair and onto your feet if possible.

Sway as in the previous exercise.
Circle your arms over your head, travelling round to the right.

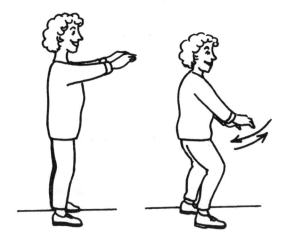

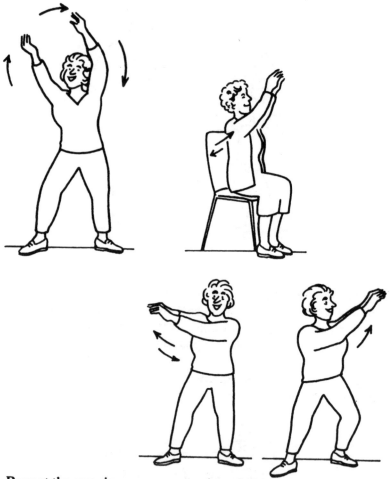

Repeat the swaying movements, then circle your arms over your head, travelling round to the left this time.

Easy walking

Use this exercise to get your breath back.

Sit or stand tall with your feet close together.
Lift one heel and then the other, taking the weight slowly from one foot to the other in a pedalling movement, distributing the weight evenly between your feet as you do so.

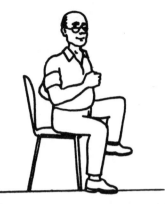

Build up to a pacy foot-pedalling speed and pump your arms forwards and back in the opposite direction to your legs.

Room walking
Walk round the room transferring the weight evenly as in the previous exercise.

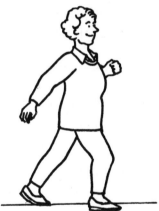

Build up to a vigorous walking rhythm, lengthening your stride, swinging your arms.
Vary the speed in bursts to get the circulation going.

Marching and rocking baby
Standing tall, march on the spot, swinging your arms in the

opposite direction to your legs, building up to a moderately vigorous marching action.

Do this briefly on the spot, then travel in a circle.

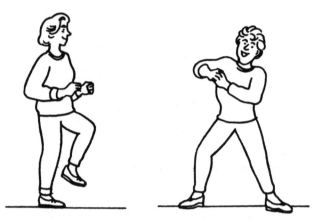

Lift your knees as you march.

Every now and again, march your feet out until they are shoulder width apart, then march in this position.

Then stand with your feet shoulder width apart and sway from side to side, swinging your arms as if rocking a baby to sleep. Swing quite a long way with control from side to side until your muscles feel warm.

Finish with some more marching in a circle, lifting your knees and swinging your arms as before.

Torvill and Dean

Pretend you are ice skating, bending your knees, transferring your weight from one leg to the other and swinging your arms across your body. Bend more deeply and push more forcefully with your legs than you did during the warm-up session.

Remember to bring these actions down gradually until you are back to an easy stage before going on to Block 5.

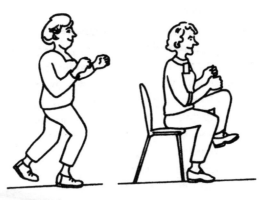

Block 5 – Cool down: mobilizing and stretching

Choose some mobilizer exercises and stretches from Block 2 and do these gently for five minutes. Then do some relaxation to complete your workout.

For suggestions for aerobic activities that are enjoyable and beneficial to your health and that you can do in addition to the exercises given in this chapter, see Chapter 4.

How to relax

Learning how to relax is an important part of managing your life, with or without arthritis but especially with. As mentioned earlier, stress makes it harder to cope with pain, so you can make the pain easier to manage if you can find effective ways to relax your body and your mind.

Research has shown that several very useful things happen to your body when you relax totally. Your pulse and breathing rates slow down, you use less oxygen, and high blood pressure drops to normal levels. The brain is also affected. When your brain is busy and active, beta waves are recorded, but when you are truly relaxed, alpha, and, sometimes, in periods of very deep relaxation, very slow theta waves interplay. Alpha and theta waves refresh and restore your body and mind.

Relaxation techniques

You can practise relaxation techniques at any time, but best of all is first thing in the morning, before breakfast, as this prepares you for the day, or last thing at night, at least two hours after your evening meal, before you go to bed, as this improves the quality of your sleep. However, you can also relax very effectively after your exercise sessions or at any other time during the day. When you get really good, you can use the techniques on a catnap basis, whenever you need extra energy.

No equipment is needed, but most people find that they relax best in a peaceful environment where there is very little noise, light or other people to distract them. Unplugging the telephone is a good idea. If this is not possible then cover it with cushions to muffle the noise. Some people find that they can ignore outside noise and can even relax effectively on a noisy commuter train or in the office during the lunch hour with phones ringing, while others will be disturbed by the slightest sound. You will know best what you can cope with, so arrange things accordingly. You will also improve with practice and find that it is well worth working at.

You need to be comfortable. You do not have to lie on the floor to relax – you can sit cross-legged or on your bed, your favourite armchair, even a straight-backed chair, anywhere as long as you can feel at ease, ideally for 10 to 20 minutes but even two minutes is better than nothing! You may also like to choose an object to concentrate on, such as a lighted candle, a flower, or a simple diagram or pattern. Position this in front of you. Alternatively, you can use a thought, a word, a prayer, the sound of birds singing, a tape of waves breaking on the sea shore, a clock ticking, your own breathing, or anything else rhythmical that appeals to you.

Before you start your relaxation session, make sure you are physically at ease. This means doing all the things that might later distract you, such as going to the toilet, blowing your nose so that you can breathe easily, changing into loose-fitting clothes, warming the room or letting in some fresh air, having a drink.

EXERCISE, REST AND RELAXATION

When you are ready, start by breathing easily – in through the nose, out through the mouth. Maintain this type of even, rhythmical, gentle breathing throughout the session. You may find it helpful to count your breaths from one to ten each time you breathe out. This is particularly useful if you have a lot of distracting thoughts. Alternatively, you can fill your mind with a visualization of your breath, following its course through your nose, down the larynx, into your lungs and out again.

Next, work towards there being no thoughts in your head other than those around your meditation object. Of course, it takes time for you to be able to do this and, at first, thoughts of all kinds will crowd into this conveniently empty space. Do not fight them – let them come and let them go and return your concentration to your chosen object.

Some people find it easier to achieve a state of full relaxation if they do a guided series of movements. For example, you can start with your hands, then move on to your arms, shoulders, upper body, lower body, thighs, knees, feet, neck and face, tensing each part then relaxing it so that you can feel the difference.

To start with you will probably find it easiest to aim to relax for about three to four minutes, but, with practice, you will find you can extend this to ten minutes and beyond. Do not worry if you fall asleep – you obviously need the rest – but continue the relaxation session when you wake. It is important to allow time at the end of the session to begin moving again. Gradually get your body up and going with some gentle mobilizing and allow the benefits you have received to drift on into the next thing you are doing. You will find that your movements will be slower and you will feel more at peace.

4

Other Forms of Exercise
You Can Do

The exercise routines given in the previous chapter, if done regularly and followed by rest, will help you to better health. Hopefully you will find that exercise is quite irresistible and, as you begin to feel fitter and more agile, you will want to do other activities, too. These will further improve your overall fitness and, equally important, be really enjoyable.

Choosing what to do

Some activities are not recommended if you have arthritis, simply because they can exacerbate your joint problems. Anything that involves sudden, violent movements, and is impact based, such as squash, tennis, or intense jogging, can do more damage to your joints. You should also avoid any exercises that involve kneeling or jumping.

When you have chosen an activity, or more than one, try not to be too enthusiastic when you start. It's easy to overstretch yourself because there is always a temptation to do that bit more, go that bit further beyond your capacity, especially if you enjoy what you are doing or are determined to improve. Remember, your body may have become very unfit while you have been coping with the arthritis. Even people *without* joint problems run the risk of injury if they overdo things, and, of course, with arthritis you are even more vulnerable.

Do not let this put you off trying something new, though, as there are many activities you *can* enjoy and that will enhance the work you are doing in the exercises given in the previous chapter. Some activities are an extension of these exercises, such as swimming, aqua exercise or walking, while others offer something quite different, say, t'ai chi. Some are more active and demanding, such as cycling, whereas others allow you to extend your range through gentle movements, for example, yoga. The choice is yours, just bear in mind the above safety guidelines.

Many people take up new activities, but large numbers drop out shortly afterwards. Once you have made the decision that exercise is going to be an essential part of your life, you need to ask yourself a few questions before starting an activity if you are to avoid joining the drop-outs!

- How accessible is it? Can you take part as often and as easily as you intend. The easier it is to get there and the more convenient the timing, the more likely you are to keep doing it.
- Will you have to travel far? Some people find it a lot easier to stick with a new interest if it is just down the road – at least there is no excuse not to go because of bad weather or the car breaking down.
- Does it fit into your life and the time you have available? If you lead a busy life and choose an activity that takes a lot of time either to get to or do, then you may find you cannot continue to fit it in.
- Is it expensive? If you need to invest in any special equipment or the cost of lessons, you need to feel committed.
- Is it dependent on the weather? If you choose something that you can only do on dry days, then you may want to look for alternatives for when the weather is against you.
- Will you meet other people? This is important for some people who like to exercise with others for encouragement and the fun of the social side.

The secret of success is to choose something that you enjoy doing, something that leaves you feeling fulfilled, refreshed, and happy afterwards, rather than exhausted and frustrated. You do not have to commit yourself to just one activity. You can, if you have the time or if it is easy to organize, do two or three. For instance, you might choose to go swimming one day, walk on two others, and take a t'ai chi class at the weekend. After several weeks, you may find that there is a single activity that you prefer and want to concentrate on or you may be happy to continue with a variety of activities.

What you choose will depend on what is available in your area and how advanced your arthritis is. The following pages will guide you through some of the likely options to help you make your own choices. Remember, though, that whatever you choose:

- before you start the activity, have a medical check-up and ask your doctor if it is suitable for you
- stop if you feel any pain and get advice before continuing
- always do a warm-up and cool-down session (use the exercises from the previous chapter) before you start and to end any exercise session
- check that your teacher is fully qualified
- progress slowly.

For addresses of associations and so on to contact to find out more about the activities described in this chapter, see Chapter 5.

Walking

The benefits of walking are well known. For many people with arthritis, it can be an ideal activity. It allows you to exercise the main muscles of the body – most of them in the legs, but remember to swing your arms, too. Doing a good warm-up before you go will ensure that all the muscles are pliable, and make it easier and safer for you to get into a good walking rhythm. It is important to do some cool-down exercises at the end of the walk as this will help avoid fatigue and stiffness and return your muscles to their normal length.

There is very little risk of injury while walking, provided that you take things slowly and do not do too much too soon. It is sensible, as you reach the end of the walk, to slow the pace until you are strolling. Then, do your cool-down and, if there is time, when you get home, some deep relaxation.

Walking is less strenuous than other aerobic activities, but once you get into a good rhythm of brisk walking, you can burn up as many calories in an hour as during a fast, 20-minute swim. It is also worth remembering that if you walk briskly for half an hour three to four times a week, you will improve your overall fitness and considerably reduce the risks of heart disease, obesity, diabetes, osteoporosis, stroke and certain cancers.

If you have done little or no exercise up until now or if your joints are painful, then you will want to take things slowly. Walking for perhaps ten minutes at a time to start with and building up to an hour over a period of weeks is a good idea. However, even if you cannot walk for this length of time, the little you do is still doing you good.

You may also feel more comfortable if you alternate the speed you walk at. Walk briskly for a while, then slowly for a bit and so on, until you feel comfortable walking briskly all the time.

Where you walk is up to you. You may prefer to use your car or bike to get to the nearest park or country path, but many people find it much easier to keep to a regular walking routine if they simply walk out of the front door and round the block.

You do not need any equipment for walking, apart from a pair of comfortable shoes – the best you can afford. They should give you good support all round and have a cushioned sole. You may want to use extra inner soles as additional shock absorbers, particularly if you will be walking on hard pavements.

Swimming and aqua exercise

Water is a perfect medium for anyone with arthritis. The support it gives the body can make it possible to do movements that are out of the question on dry land. Swimming is an excellent aerobic exercise that improves three major areas of fitness: mobility and flexibility, muscle endurance, and aerobic fitness. Unlike other forms of exercise, it does allow you to use *all* your muscles, and the more strokes you do, the greater the variety of movements you will put your muscles through. Because water cushions your body, the risk of injury is much reduced.

OTHER FORMS OF EXERCISE YOU CAN DO

As well as simply swimming lengths or widths, you may be able to try aqua exercise. When you exercise in water, you may feel as if you are not doing much, but, in fact, you will be achieving a great deal.

You can try marching, first on the spot while holding onto the side and then, if you feel confident, moving through the water. Wrist- and ankle-mobilizing exercises can also be done in water – in the bath as well as in the pool. If you wish to exercise in a pool, it is a good idea to do this with a friend who can offer encouragement and support. If you feel at all unsteady in the water, it is perfectly acceptable to wear arm bands, rubber rings or use polystyrene floats for support – although remember that these do not take the place of life jackets if you are in the sea.

The alternative is to join an aqua exercise class. Most public swimming pools and leisure centres offer these, but make sure before you sign on that you have chosen a session that is right for you. Some, which combine swimming and aerobics, are quite demanding. The teacher should be properly trained in aqua exercise and be able to advise you on what exercises to leave out if they are likely to exacerbate your condition.

If your arthritis is particularly bad, you may be able to have sessions in a hydrotherapy pool. Your GP should be able to arrange this. Often these will be supervised by a physiotherapist who will give you movements to do as well as help you into and out of the pool. The water in a hydrotherapy pool is a great deal warmer than that in the average public pool (usually over 90 degrees) and this makes it easier to relax and really enjoy the feeling of being able to move with ease.

For many people, swimming is an ideal form of exercise. The only likely drawback is that, unless the pool is very close, it may be difficult to go three or four times a week. This is why people often combine swimming with other activities. Also, it can become very monotonous simply swimming lengths. Try using different strokes and meditation techniques, such as counting strokes, repeating a word or phrase or simply concentrating on the movements of your body so that you benefit mentally as well as physically.

Cycling

This can be a relatively safe form of exercise for most people with arthritis. The non-weight-bearing pedalling movements do not jar the joints, although the constant repetition of movement involved may make cycling unsuitable for you if you have trouble with your hips or knees.

Cycling is enjoyable if the road is flat, there is little or no traffic, and you are in the country, but if you live in a town or a hilly area, it may be less pleasurable and less suitable.

Again, you need to start slowly, choosing a short, flat route, building up to something more demanding as and when you feel ready. Doing warm-up exercises before and cool-down exercises afterwards is essential.

If you are thinking of buying a bike, remember that mountain bikes are good for off-road cycling, but are heavy to carry, and to pedal on the road, the standard touring bike suits most people, while a lightweight racing bike is wonderfully light to carry and makes hills a lot easier. Make sure the bike is the right size for your height. The most important measurement is the distance from the pedal to the saddle, which should be a little more than the length of your inside leg.

Cycling can be a very sociable form of exercise, too. Most areas have a branch of the Cyclists' Touring Club, where you can meet other enthusiasts.

Yoga

If you are looking for other ways to improve your flexibility and muscle strength, then yoga is a good choice. As well as helping your muscles, yoga will also help you to improve your breath control, and, through practising the different positions (asanas), you learn to release tension. Yoga is completely non-competitive. Each person does the asanas to the best of their ability, never straining or overstretching.

Each session starts with a period of relaxation and ends with a meditation, which can be done lying down or sitting, whichever feels most comfortable to you. Because the movements are done so carefully and slowly, they are ideal if you have arthritis as they will help improve strength and flexibility without straining the joints. However, certain yoga positions such as the plough, neck and hand circles, and the bow, are now recognized as being unsound if you have arthritis, so you should not do them. The meditation can help you to feel more at peace with yourself and the way you are.

Many of the asanas for beginners are simple, so you can practise them at home on your own, but joining a class to start with gives you a better idea of what it is all about. A good yoga teacher will be aware of current thinking, aware of the needs of their pupils, help you to do as much as is comfortable, and make sure you avoid any exercise that could hurt your joints, such as those involving kneeling.

Alexander Technique

This teaches you how to improve your posture. After a series of lessons. You will stand and move better, and with more purpose. This could be especially useful if you suffer a lot of pain as a result of tension.

It is not possible to learn the Alexander Technique from a book. You need to go to a trained teacher who will be able to show you how to establish the right co-ordination between your neck, head and back. You can then go home and gradually introduce what you have been taught into your daily life.

Feldenkrais method

Feldenkrais is similar to the Alexander Technique in that it too aims to re-educate you about the way you move.

Feldenkrais concentrates on the mastering of very small movements and most exercises are done on the floor. The result is better posture, and it can also reduce the amount of wear and tear on the joints – an important point if you have arthritis.

T'ai chi ch'uan

T'ai chi is a series of slow, flowing, rhythmic movements. It is very gentle, yet, as well as strengthening muscles, it will help you to develop better balance and co-ordination. Again, you need to go to a class to learn the movements, which you can then practise at home.

As with yoga, a whole philosophy and approach to life is attached to t'ai chi. You do not have to take this on board in order to do the movements, but you may find that, gradually, your attitudes and feelings are changing.

Working out

Most leisure centres offer a choice of circuit training, multi-gyms, weights, and classes in Step and other kinds of exercise. Most have the latest equipment and you can tailor things to your needs and level of fitness. Some of the equipment may be quite useful for you. For instance, you may be able to have sessions on an exercise bike there rather than going to the expense of buying one of your own.

Before using any of the equipment, though, you should have a proper fitness assessment from a member of staff at the centre who is qualified to do this. You will be shown round and advised about what equipment to use and what to avoid, depending on which joints are affected. An individual programme of exercise should be devised for you, which you can build on over the coming weeks and months.

5

Where to Find Out More

Support and information

Arthritis Care, 18 Stephenson Way, London NW1 2HD
Tel.: 020 7380 6500 Helpline: 0808 800 4050 (10 a.m.–
4 p.m. weekdays only)   Website: www.arthritiscare.org.uk
For information and advice on all aspects of arthritis. There
are local branches nationwide, and Young Arthritis Care (for
anybody with arthritis who is under 45) has its own groups,
local contacts, magazine and online resources at www.
arthritiscare.org.uk/LivingwithArthritis/Youngpeople

Arthritis Research UK, Copeman House, St Mary's
Court, St Mary's Gate, Chesterfield, Derbyshire S41 7TD
Tel.: 0300 790 0400   Website: www.arthritisresearchuk.org

Backcare, 16 Elmtree Road, Teddington, Middlesex TW11 8ST
Helpline: 0845 130 2704   Website: www.backcare.org.uk

Lupus UK, St James House, Eastern Road, Romford, Essex
RM1 3NH
Tel.: 01708 731251   Email: headoffice@lupus.org.uk
Website: www.lupusuk.org.uk

The Margaret Hills Clinic, 1 Oaks Precinct, Caesar Road,
Kenilworth, Warwickshire CV8 1DP. Tel.: 01926 854783
Website: www.margarethillsclinic.com
Send a stamped addressed envelope for information and
advice on the natural treatment of arthritis.

National Osteoporosis Society, Camerton, Bath BA2 OPJ.
Tel: 01761 471771   Helpline: 0845 450 0230
Email: info@nos.org.uk   Website: www.nos.org.uk

Scoliosis Association (UK), 2 Ivebury Court, 325 Latimer
Road, London W10 6RA
Tel.: 020 8964 5343   Helpline: 020 8964 1166
Email: sauk@sauk.org.uk   Website: www.sauk.org.uk

How you can help yourself

One of the more important things that you will probably have learned as a result of having arthritis is that you want to protect and comfort your inflamed and damaged joints as much as possible. There are several things that you can do to make life easier and relieve some of the stress on your joints:

- unless rest is essential, try not to stay in one position for too long, and when you are sitting, adjust your position quite frequently so that joints do not become locked. When you are driving, stop at least every hour for a break
- learn how to use your back properly, always bending from the knees to pick things up
- make your life efficient if you can by cutting down on the number of tasks you do around the house. For instance, let the washing-up drain and dry, and when you pick anything up, use both hands if this feels easier.

There are many items available that can help make life easier and it makes sense to look at them rather than struggling to cope without them as this can only increase tension and pain. Some examples include the following. There are particularly strong shopping trolleys available that have a seat. They can be used for support and will not tip up. To avoid bending, there are many types of reacher, some with magnetic tips, to help you pick things up off the floor without bending, and long-handled brushes and combs. There are kettle tippers so that you can pour without having to lift the kettle. If your grip is weak, try broad-handled cutlery, fat pens, and handles for keys and plugs, tap turners, and handles for turning knobs.

In the bathroom you can overcome problems with getting into and out of the bath by installing grab rails or by getting a bath insert. In the bedroom, make sure your bed is comfortable and look at the range of equipment that can make time spent in bed easier, such as pillow supports and book rests.

For the garden, you get long-handled, lightweight tools, and special kneeling stools. The Society for Horticultural Therapy (now registered as Thrive, and based at the Geoffrey Udall Centre, Beech Hill, Reading RG7 2AT: tel.: 0118 988 5688) can answer queries; visit the websites www.thrive.org.uk and www.carryongardening.org.uk for more information.

In short, there are very few areas of life that cannot be made easier for you with the right aid or piece of equipment. Some items can be provided free of charge by your local authority, most can be bought, and some can be hired.

All over the country, there are Disabled Living Centres where, if you make an appointment, you can see quite a wide variety of aids and try them for yourself. For details of your nearest centre, contact Disabled Living Centres, Redbank House, 4 St Chad's Street, Cheetham, Manchester M8 8QA; tel: 0161 214 5959; website: www.disabledliving.co.uk. The Disabled Living Foundation is also a good source of information and advice; tel.: 020 7289 6111; helpline 0845 130 9177, 10 a.m. to 4 p.m., Mondays to Fridays; website: www.dlf.org.uk

Founded in 1977 as the Royal Association for Disability and Rehabilitation, RADAR: The Disability Network produces a number of useful leaflets and much else for disabled people (12 City Forum, 250 City Road, London EC1V 8AF; tel: 020 7250 3222, 10 a.m. to 4 p.m., Mondays to Fridays; website: www.radar.org.uk. Remap, D9 Chaucer Business Park, Kemsing, Sevenoaks, Kent TN15 6YU; tel.: 0845 130 0456; website: www.remap.org.uk, can provide 'one-off' items if the aid or equipment you need is not commercially available.

Various companies also have a good range of aids to independent living. Boots publish an 'Active and Independent' catalogue, available free from large branches or by contacting Boots Customer Care, PO Box 5300, Nottingham NG90 1AA (tel.: 0845 609 0055). You can also obtain useful catalogues from:

- Hearing and Mobility (branches all over the country), Unit 3/4 Sterling Park, Pedmore Road, Brierley Hill, West Midlands DY5 1TB, tel.: 0844 888 1338; website: www.hearingandmobility.co.uk

- The Special Collection, J. D. Williams, Griffin House, 40 Lever Street, Manchester M60 6ES, tel.: 0871 231 2000; website: www.specialcollection.com
- You're Able offers various products to help with daily living (Nunn Brook Road, Huthwaite, Sutton-in-Ashfield, Notts NG17 2HU; tel.: 01632 448703; website: www.youreableshop.co.uk

Products that help relieve pain

As well as your active involvement in dealing with the pain your arthritis causes by changes in your diet and lifestyle and doing exercise, there are some products you can use that may help relieve pain and, in some cases, make it possible for you to do more exercise to improve things.

Most physiotherapists will recommend ice or heat packs to place on inflamed joints. You can also buy battery-operated vibration cushions and, when these are placed against the back, shoulder or knee, they may ease the pain.

TENS machines help some people and if your doctor can refer you to a local pain clinic you can be taught various ways to help cope with the pain.

The bath is often a place where you can find relief. Spa baths are an expensive option but do bring relief for many. Margaret Hills recommends an air bubble massage bath, which is invaluable for improving the cirulation, helps to relieve stress and tension and can massage specific areas of the body, such as the feet, bust, hips, knees, and back. For further details about this bath, write to the Margaret Hills Clinic (see page 94).

Alternative therapies

Some arthritis sufferers have found additional relief through alternative therapies. There are many to choose from, but treatment is unlikely to be available on the NHS. It is important to go to a qualified therapist and the best way to find one local to you is to approach the organization that represents the therapy.

Here are a few you might like to try:

- Association of Reflexologists, 5 Fore Street, Taunton, Somerset TA1 1HX; tel.: 01823 351010; website www.aor.org.uk
- British Acupuncture Council, 63 Jeddo Road, London W12 9HQ; tel: 020 8735 0400; www.acupuncture.org.uk
- British Chiropractic Association, 59 Castle Street, Reading, Berkshire RG1 7SN; tel.: 0118 950 5950; website: www.chiropractic-uk.co.uk
- British Complementary Medicine Association, PO Box 5122, Bournemouth BH8 0WG; tel.: 0845 345 5977; website: www.bcma.co.uk (represents a large number of complementary therapists and runs a referral scheme to help find a registered practitioner in your area).
- The British Homeopathic Association represents medically qualified homeopaths (Hahnemann House, 29 Park Street West, Luton LU1 3BE; tel: 01582 408675; website: www.britishhomeopathic.org. Also see the Society of Homeopaths, 11 Brookfield, Duncan Close, Moulton Park, Northampton NN3 6WL; tel: 0845 450 6611; website: www.homeopathy-soh.org
- General Osteopathic Council, 176 Tower Bridge Road, London SE1 3LU; tel.: 020 7357 6655; Website: www.osteopathy.org.uk
- General Regulatory Council for Complementary Therapies, Swift House, High Street, Stavely, Chesterfield S43 3UX; tel.: 0870 3144031; website: www.grcct.org. They can provide information on practitioners of complementary therapies, including aromatherapists.
- Institute for Complementary and Natural Medicine, Can-Mezzanine, 32–36 Loman Street, London SE1 0EH; tel.: 020 7922 7980; website: www.i-c-m.org.uk. The institute can provide information on who best to approach among the various complementary therapies.
- The Margaret Hills Clinic (see page 94)
- Shiatsu Society UK, PO Box 4580, Rugby CV21 9EL; tel.: 0845 130 4560; website: www.shiatsusociety.org

Two excellent books to read to find out ways to manage pain are: Neville Shone's *Coping Successfully With Pain* (Sheldon Press, revised edition 2002) and Margaret Hills' *Treating Arthritis: The drug-free way* (Sheldon Press, revised edition 2004), which also includes advice about all aspects of arthritis.

Exercise and activities

Walking

The Ramblers Association, 2nd Floor, Camelford House, 87–90 Albert Embankment, London SE1 7TW
Tel.: 020 7339 8500
Website: www.ramblers.org.uk

Cycling

Bicycle Association, 3 the Quadrant, Coventry CV1 2DY
Tel.: 02476 553838
Website: www.ba-gb.com

Cyclists' Touring Club (CTC), Parklands, Railton Road, Guildford, Surrey GU2 9JX
Tel: 0844 736 8450
Website: www.ctc.org.uk

Yoga

British Wheel of Yoga, 25 Jermyn Street, Sleaford, Lincolnshire NG34 7RU
Tel: 01529 306851
Website: www.bwy.org.uk

Iyengar Yoga Institute, 223a Randolph Avenue, London W9 1NL
Tel.: 020 7624 3080
Website: www.iyi.org.uk

Yoga for Health and Education Trust, 24 Brighton Terrace, Todmorden, Lancs OL14 8LA (membership enquiries); 18 Haymarket, Lytham St Annes FY8 3LW (all other enquiries)
Website: www.yoga-health-education.org.uk

Alexander Technique

Alexander Technique International, UK Regional Coordinator, Graham Elliott, 28 Marshal's Drive, St Albans, Herts AL1 4RQ
Tel.: 01727 760 067
Website: www.ati-met.com

The website lists branches around the world.

Society of Teachers of the Alexander Technique, 1st Floor, Linton House, 39–51 Highgate Road, London NW5 1RS
Tel.: 020 7482 5135
Website: www.stat.org.uk

Feldenkrais

The Feldenkrais Guild UK, Scott Clark, 13 Camellia House, Idonia Street, London SE8 4LZ
Tel.: 07000 785 506
Website: www.feldenkrais.co.uk

T'ai chi

The T'ai Chi Union for Great Britain, Ronnie Robinson (Publicity), 1 Littlemill Drive, Balmoral Gardens, Crookston, Glasgow G53 7GF
Website: www.taichiunion.com

Working out

Extend Exercise Training Ltd, 2 Place Farm, Wheathampstead, Herts AL4 8SB
Tel.: 01582 832760
Website: www.extend.org.uk

A charity providing movement-to-music classes for over-60s and people of all ages with disabilities; there are teachers all over the country. For your nearest, telephone or visit the website.

Medau Movement, 1 Grove House, Foundry Lane, Horsham, W. Sussex RH13 5PL
Tel.: 01403 266000
Website: www.medau.org.uk

Index